Second Edition

BABIES
with DOWN
SYNDROME

A New Parents' Guide
Edited by Karen Stray-Gundersen

WOODBINE HOUSE • 1995

Figure 2 in Chapter 6 reprinted by permission of Siegfried M. Pueschel, M.D., Ph.D., M.P.H. and Andrews, McMeel and Parker from *Down Syndrome: Growing and Learning (1978)*. All rights reserved.

Cover Illustration: Annie Lunsford
Photographs: Gayle Krughoff, National Down Syndrome Congress, and parents

Library of Congress Cataloging-in-Publication Data

Babies with Down syndrome : a new parents' guide / edited by Karen Stray-Gundersen. — 2nd ed.
    p.   cm.
   Includes bibliographical references and index.
   ISBN-13: 978-0-933149-64-9
   ISBN-10: 0-933149-64-6
   1. Down's syndrome—Popular works. 2. Mentally handicapped children—Care. I. Stray-Gundersen, Karen.
RJ506.D68B33 1995   95-34041
618.92'858842—dc20   CIP

Manufactured in the United States of America

15 14 13

With deep affection and admiration, this book
is dedicated to babies with Down syndrome
and their parents.

TABLE OF CONTENTS

Foreword

Ann M. Forts*

Hi! My name is Ann Margaret Forts and I do not have "Down" syndrome. I really am an "UP" syndrome person, and I really love my life. I have lots and lots of friends. My life is very busy with all kinds of activities. Some things I can do very well while others not so good. Anyway, the important thing is that I always try my best and I really enjoy what I do. I guess that's because I do get lots of encouragement from my family and friends.

I think it is time for everyone to start thinking "UP" instead of "Down." I wish the name of the doctor who discovered Down syndrome was Dr. Up instead of Dr. Down. Then maybe more people would start with a better attitude toward us than they do now. Maybe they would understand what we are all about and what we are capable of doing.

Sometimes I meet people who make me very unhappy because they think they know everything and won't give me a chance to prove myself. I enjoy showing them that they are

---

* Ann M. Forts is a member of the Board of Directors of the National Down Syndrome Congress; the New Hampshire Developmental Disabilities Council; and the President's Committee on Mental Retardation. She is the Editor-in-Chief of *Down Syndrome Headline News*, a publication of the National Down Syndrome Congress by and for people with Down syndrome. Ann's favorite work is public speaking all over the United States as a self-advocate and motivational speaker at meetings, conferences, and workshops for parent support organizations, professionals, schools & colleges, and civic organizations. She also works as a hostess at a gourmet restaurant, a video rental store clerk, and a supermarket bagger. In 1995, Ann was chosen to receive a new international award called the "Self Empowerment Award," from the Joseph P. Kennedy, Jr. Foundation for her work on behalf of people with mental retardation. In her spare time, Ann enjoys water and snow skiing, traveling, and playing with her eight nieces and nephews.

wrong—in fact, very wrong. I don't think it is fair for anyone to tell me that I am not capable of doing or learning something, especially when they don't give me a chance to try.

If people want to help us, they really should try lots of encouragement, guidance, and patience. For our part, we should always try our best; take pride in what we do; try to meet new people and make lots of friends; speak for ourselves; learn to be independent; and try new experiences. Then we will be able to make things happen for ourselves rather than waiting for someone else to do things for us. Then we will be on the "UP" side of "Down" syndrome.

Congratulations to all you parents of a new baby with Down Syndrome! I can tell you from my personal experience that your baby can and will develop into a really "UP" person, especially if *you* stay on the "UP" side of Down Syndrome. Then there will be many times that you will have the satisfaction of hearing your child say my favorite expression: "I love my life!"

Staying on the "UP" side of Down Syndrome means many things like lots of love; patience; kindness; encouragement; being proud of us; helping us to be independent; giving us a chance to succeed or even sometimes allowing us to experience failure. Always believe in us, encourage us, and, even if at times it takes us a little longer to do what we are trying to do, you will be surprised at what we will be able to do by ourselves. Don't ever try to set limits on what we are able to do because I can guarantee that you will guess wrong and that we will surprise you with our accomplishments.

My best wishes to you all for an exciting, challenging, and satisfying life with your new "UP" baby. "UP" with Down Syndrome!

Introduction

When our little boy was born, my husband and I were told they wanted to test his chromosomes; the doctors said they wanted to check for "Trisomy 21." We suspected that we should be worried about something, but didn't know what; we didn't know that Trisomy 21 meant Down syndrome. A few days later we knew.

Our first image was a desperate one, primarily because we had literally no information or knowledge of what Down syndrome was. We expected the worst. We immediately tried to learn more about Down syndrome, but found little to read. What we did find was a collection of outdated and often insensitive material. But over time we learned a lot—mostly from doctors, teachers, Down syndrome organizations, other parents, and of course, our son, with whom we fell madly in love.

This book was originally compiled to provide new parents with a complete introduction to Down syndrome. We hoped to help other parents avoid the time we spent searching for information and worrying over inaccuracies. We intended to provide you, the parent, with what we missed: up-to-date facts about what Down syndrome is and information about how to start dealing with it. Most importantly, we wanted to tell you that kids with Down syndrome are kids first and foremost. Once you understand Down syndrome you can get on to loving your new baby.

Since the first edition of this book was published, nine years have passed. Our son is now almost twelve, and our family has continued to grow. In addition to his older sister, he now has two younger brothers. In those nine years, he has gone to school and he has learned to read, write, and ride a bike. He has friends, he likes to watch movies, and he loves his dog. In short, he has blended in with the rest of our family.

During those nine years, many things for children with Down syndrome have improved. There are better educational opportunities, better health care practices, and better laws to protect the rights of our children. However, there is still a lot of outdated and inaccurate information about Down syndrome. We still think that there is a need for the basic introduction to Down syndrome our book provides. That is why we have produced a new edition. We hope you find it useful.

The chapters in this book cover the full range of things you need to start thinking about for your baby's early years—from birth to about age five or six. They explain what Down syndrome is, how to cope with the fact that your baby has Down syndrome, and how to deal with potential medical concerns. Those are the basics; from there you need information on daily care, your family life, your baby's development and education, and finally, your baby's legal rights. Each of these important subjects is covered in the book. Children with Down syndrome present great challenges, and even greater rewards. This book will help you to see your baby's great potential.

A special part of this book is its Parent Statements at the end of each chapter. In them parents who have gone through what you are going through now share their experiences, thoughts, and advice. You will find that every parent has a different slant on the same problem or experience. Combining the Parent Statements with the basic information in each chapter gives the book a real-life perspective.

You cannot do it alone and you don't need to. This book contains an extensive Resource Guide that has been updated for this edition. It will help you get in touch with parents like yourself, with doctors, teachers, therapists, and other professionals, with federal, state, and local government agencies, and with a variety of organizations that can give you the support and information you need. This book gives you the facts you need to take full advantage of the programs and services available to help your child.

Down syndrome has its own language, and parents need to learn it to best help their baby. At the end of this book is a glossary of key terms. There is also an updated and revised Reading List with books the authors and the editor recommend for further reading for new parents.

Our book also contains photographs of children with Down syndrome, at play, at home, and at school. Most of the children are age three and under.

No book can mend a broken heart or shattered dreams. But it can give you the facts you need to begin dreaming once again of the bright future all parents want for their children.

Throughout the book we use the personal pronouns alternately by chapter. We felt uncomfortable referring only to either boys or girls, and felt that constantly using "he or she" to refer to children would be unwieldy. When the references are to the parents and professionals, we were able to use both pronouns because it happened less frequently. Hopefully this arrangement will be clear.

This book is obviously the combined effort of many people. Each chapter was written by a parent or professional highly respected in their field. Each was motivated by a desire to inform people about the reality of Down syndrome. We gratefully acknowledge their generous contribution, In addition, we would like to thank the following people for their contribution and support in our efforts: Lawrence Cohen, M.D., Gena Daggett, Maureen Flanagan, Seymour Hepner, M.D., Marshall Keys, M.D., Kenneth Rosenbaum, M.D., Kathy Rodriguez, and Ruth Wells. Both the National Down Syndrome Congress and the National Information Center for Children and Youth with Disabilities provided essential information and assistance for the book, and we would like to express our appreciation. Our sincere thanks also go to Susan Stokes and Marshall Levin for their fine work on the book's manuscript.

We owe a special thanks to the many parents who allowed us to interview them and to photograph their beautiful children. Lastly, we want to thank all those people—parents and professionals alike—who shared their lives out of a deep commitment to help babies and their parents.

All children require care and hard work. Children with Down syndrome do too. Raising any child can be very rewarding; raising a child with Down syndrome will be equally rewarding. Your baby will never quit on himself, and you won't quit on him either. He will always try to please you and will work extremely hard during lessons and therapy. He will inspire you to do the same in learning, teaching, and advocating for him. And as you work, live, and play with your child, you will fall in love.

Everyone associated with this book wishes you a happy and fulfilling life with your new baby.

Karen Stray-Gundersen
September 1995

One

⌇⌇⌇⌇⌇

What Is Down Syndrome?

Chahira Kozma, M.D.*

The best way to understand Down syndrome—what it means to your baby and what it means to you—is to get the facts. For a condition that has for so long been shrouded in fear and darkness, the facts are far better than the myths. The worst enemy facing parents of babies with Down syndrome is ignorance. Before you do anything or decide anything about your baby, learn about Down syndrome.

This chapter introduces you to Down syndrome even if you have never heard of it before or know little about it. It addresses the basic questions parents have about Down syndrome and gives the foundation of knowledge you need to begin properly caring for your baby.

No one will say that raising a child with Down syndrome is a picnic; it is not a picnic raising *any* child. The thousands of parents who have done it successfully will say that there is a lot of hard work and patience involved. But with today's medical and educational advances, the myths and stereotypes of the past that so deprived children with Down syndrome have given way to facts and rising expectations.

* Dr. Chahira Kozma is Assistant Professor of Pediatrics and a Clinical Geneticist at Georgetown University Medical Center in Washington, D.C.

What Is Down Syndrome?

If you are like most people, you probably had little understanding of what Down syndrome meant before your baby was
born. Basically, Down syndrome means that your baby has one
extra chromosome in each of his millions of cells. Instead of 46,
he has 47. Over six thousand babies with Down syndrome are
born in the United States every year and thousands more in
other countries. It occurs in boys and girls evenly. It is one of
the most common birth defects, occurring in all races, ethnic
groups, socio-economic classes, and nationalities. It can happen
to anyone.

Because chromosomes and the genetic material they carry
play a large part in determining your child's characteristics, this
extra chromosome will affect his life. His appearance may be a
bit different from other children's, he may have some unique
medical problems, and he will likely have some degree of mental retardation, although the severity of any of these problems
varies tremendously from child to child.

Two things about Down syndrome are clear. First, parents
do not cause Down syndrome; nothing you did or did not do before or during pregnancy caused your baby to have Down syndrome. Second, like "normal" children, each baby with Down
syndrome is unique, with his own personality, talents, and
thoughts. There are few absolutes governing your baby's des-
tiny; like other children, he is an individual and will grow to become a distinct personality.

Down syndrome is not the only chromosomal abnormality
that can affect children; far from it. Parents frequently are
amazed at how often abnormal chromosomes occur at conception. In general, chromosomal abnormalities of one kind or another are very common at conception. A significant number of
chromosomal abnormalities do not allow embryos to develop,
and result in spontaneous abortions (miscarriages).

Down syndrome, the most common chromosomal abnormality in humans, is one that usually does allow the embryo to develop. As mentioned before, Down syndrome occurs in all races

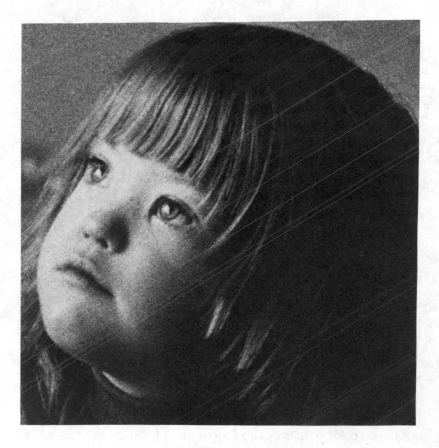

and in all countries. Recent figures place the frequency in
North America at about one in seven to eight hundred births.

What Causes Down Syndrome?

To understand what has caused your child to have Down
syndrome, you need to know something about genetics, specifically about genes and chromosomes, and about how cells divide
and grow.

Genes. Every person has genes located in every cell of the
body; they are the blueprint of life. The genes provide the cells
with instructions for growth and development. If you imagine
the human body as a computer, the genes are the software that
tells the computer what to do. Almost all of a person's traits—

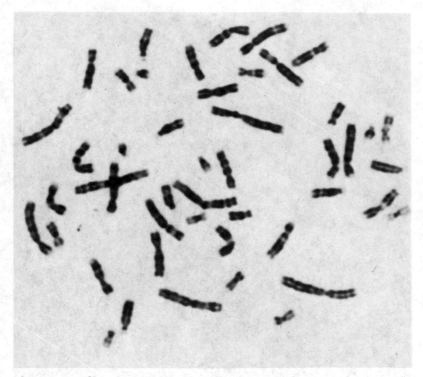

Figure 1. Chromosomes

from eye color to hand size to the sound of his voice—are coded in the genes. Every person has millions of them.

Genes are made up of a special material called DNA (deoxyribonucleic acid). In genes, DNA lines up in long strands in the shape of a twisted ladder. DNA itself is made up of long chains of molecules called *nucleotides*. The pattern and sequence of these nucleotides in the gene or DNA strand is the genetic code.

Genes come in pairs, with one member of each pair coming from the father and the other from the mother. For example, the father's genes that control hair color have their match in the mother's genes, and it is the combination of these genes that their children inherit. This combination of genes from both parents contributes to the tremendous diversity that exists among people.

Chromosomes. Genes are located on microscopic, rod-shaped bodies called chromosomes inside our cells. These are shown in Figure 1. The chromosomes are the packages that contain the genes. Usually, there are 46 chromosomes in each cell of our bodies. Chromosomes come in 23 pairs with 1 member of each pair donated by each parent via the sperm (father) or the egg cell (mother). Only one of the 23 pairs of chromosomes is created differently. These are the chromosomes that determine sex.

Cell Division. Except for the reproductive cells (eggs and sperm), all other cells in our body ordinarily contain 46 chromosomes in 23 pairs. Cells reproduce themselves through a process called *mitosis.* During mitosis the original cell (called a *parent cell*) duplicates its contents, including its chromosomes. Two *daughter cells* are produced from that one parent cell with each containing the exact 46 chromosomes of the parent. Figure 2 shows the process of mitosis. Almost all of the cells in the human body reproduce themselves through mitosis, with the important exception of the sperm and egg cells.

Sperm and egg cells are created from a different process, called *meiosis.* Meiosis works just like mitosis, except for one major difference. In meiosis, each pair of chromosomes splits or *disjoins* from each other and each daughter cell receives only one chromosome from the original pair. Before they are fully developed, reproductive cells start out with 46 chromosomes. But as they mature, meiosis reduces their chromosome count to twenty-three. Thus, at conception the sperm and egg each contain only 23 chromosomes, half the usual number. Figure 3 (page 7) shows how meiosis occurs. Errors in chromosome division during meiosis are very common. For instance, more than half of all spontaneous miscarriages during the first trimester of gestation have chromosome abnormalities. In the general population, the incidence of chromosome abnormalities is about 5 in 1,000 live births or one-half of one percent. However, in children with mental retardation and multiple birth defects, the incidence rises to between 8 and 14 percent.

Fertilization. At conception the sperm and egg cells combine, yielding one fertilized egg with a complete set of 46 chromosomes, 23 from the mother and 23 from father. Figure 4 (page 8) shows what occurs during fertilization. Soon after fertilization, the fertilized egg begins to grow and develop by dividing by mitosis into two identical new cells, and it continues mitosis until there are billions of cells. As cells duplicate, their genetic material is also duplicated so that each new cell receives the exact same chromosomal material as the original fertilized cell. Because all cells duplicate the genetic structure of that first fertilized egg, its genetic content determines the genetic makeup of the baby.

Figure 5 (page 9) shows a picture of normal chromosomes. Called *karyotypes,* these pictures are made from blood samples

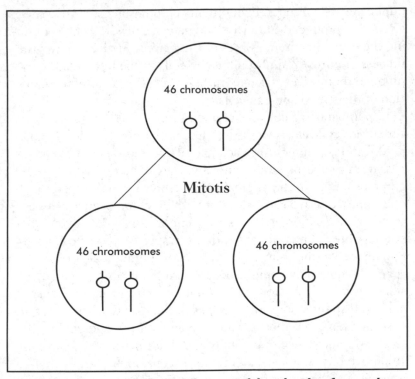

Figure 2. Mitosis: Cell division resulting in the formation of two cells, each with the same chromosome complement as the parent cell. For simplicity, only one pair of chromosomes is illustrated in all figures.

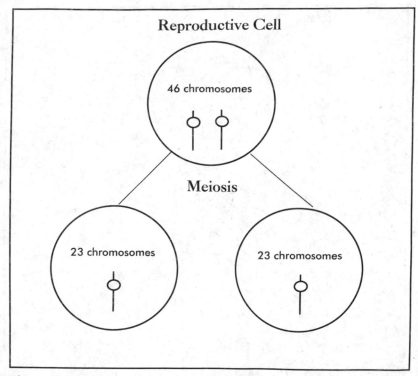

Figure 3. Meiosis: Special cell division that occurs in the reproductive call (egg and sperm) by which only one member of each pair of chromosomes goes to the daughter cell and the total chromosome count becomes 23.

taken from babies after birth. The blood samples are *cultured*—allowed to grow in a petri dish—and the chromosomes are then isolated by a microscope or camera. The chromosomes are then grouped into pairs and numbered according to their size. As you can see, there are 23 pairs of chromosomes. Chromosomes are believed to function in tandem, with each set carefully balanced. If for some reason, an extra chromosome is present, the genetic balance is thrown off.

A number of abnormal events or mistakes can occur during meiosis that can affect a child's growth and development. Some of these mistakes can lead to Down syndrome. Down syndrome

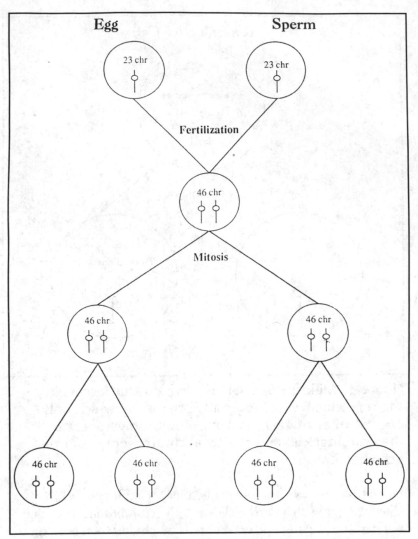

Figure 4: During fertilization, the 23 chromosomes from the egg and sperm combine. The resulting fertilized egg has 46 chromosomes.

usually results from what is called *nondisjunction*, or failure of one pair of chromosomes to separate evenly during meiosis. In nondisjunction, one daughter cell receives 24 chromosomes and the other cell 22 chromosomes. A cell with only 22 chromosomes

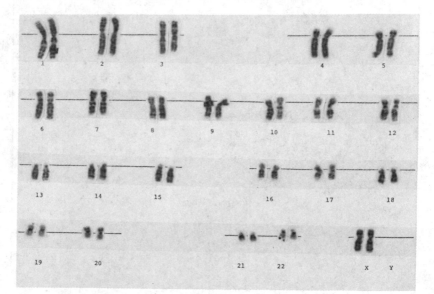

Figure 5. Karyotype of Normal Chromosomes

(missing an entire chromosome) cannot survive and cannot be fertilized. On the other hand, an egg or sperm cell with 24 chromosomes can survive and can be fertilized. When this occurs, the resulting fertilized egg has 47 chromosomes instead of the normal 46 chromosomes. Doctors refers to this condition as a *trisomy* (three chromosomes). Figure 6 (page 10) shows how nondisjunction occurs. In Down syndrome it is the number-21 chromosome that does not separate properly. This is referred to as *Trisomy 21,* which is another term for Down syndrome.

In Trisomy 21, erroneous chromosome division during meiosis results in the fertilized egg having three number-21 chromosomes instead of two. As the newly created embryo begins to grow by dividing and duplicating itself, the extra chromosome is also copied and transmitted to each new cell. The result is that all cells contain the extra number-21 chromosome. This type of Down syndrome is called *Nondisjunction Trisomy 21,* meaning it results from failure of the chromosome 21 pair to disjoin from each other or divide properly in the egg or sperm cells. Figure 7 (page 11) is a karyotype of the chromosomes of a baby with

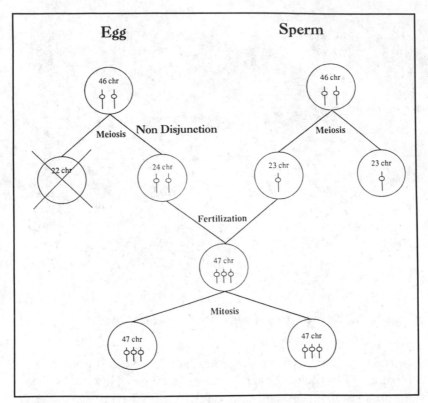

Figure 6: Nondisjunction is the failure of the pair of chromosomes to separate during meiosis resulting in both number–21 chromosomes being carried to one daughter cell and none to the other. Upon conception, the fertilized egg contains 47 chromosomes, leading to Nondisjunction Trisomy 21.

Down syndrome, and shows the extra number-21 chromosome. About 95 percent of babies with Down syndrome have Nondisjunction Trisomy 21.

The 8 percent of babies with Down syndrome who do not have Nondisjunction Trisomy 21 have one of two other types: *Translocation* or *Mosaicism.* In Translocation Trisomy 21, there are 3 copies of the number-21 chromosome. However, the extra chromosome is attached to another chromosome, usually chromosome 14 or the other number-21 chromosome. Three to four percent of babies with Down syndrome have Translocation Trisomy 21. They usually have the same characteristics as babies with Nondisjunction Trisomy 21. Figure 8 shows the karyotype of a person with Translocation Trisomy 21.

About one-fourth of translocations occur spontaneously during fertilization. This happens when a piece of a chromosome or a whole chromosome breaks off during meiosis and attaches itself to another chromosome. When the chromosome piece attaches itself (translocates) to chromosome 21, the resulting fertilized egg has Down syndrome or Translocation Trisomy 21. The other three-fourths of translocations are inherited from a parent. This is the only type of Down syndrome that can result from a condition in a parent's genes. When this happens, the carrier parent has the typical number of chromosomes, but two of his or her chromosome pairs are stuck together. As a result, their total chromosome count is 45 instead of 46. He or she is unaffected because there is no loss or excess of genetic material; just the usual amount with two chromosomes stuck together. Doctors refer to a parent like this as a *balanced carrier*. Knowing

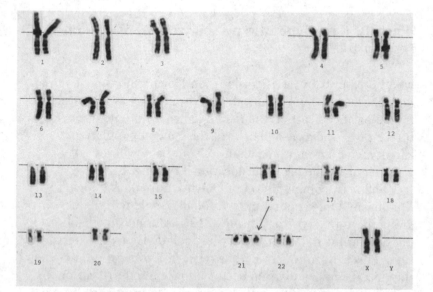

Figure 7. Karyotype of Chromosomes with Nondisjunction Trisomy 21

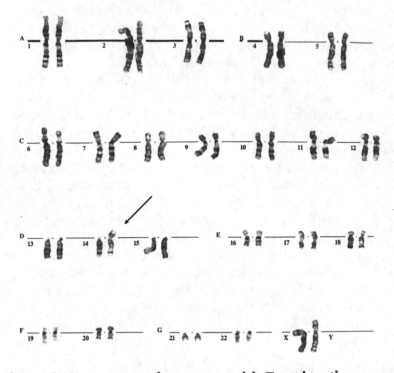

Figure 8. Karyotype of a person with Translocation Trisomy 21.

whether your baby has Translocation Down syndrome is important because if the Translocation Trisomy 21 was inherited from a balanced carrier, the risk of Down syndrome occurring in future pregnancies is higher than the general population. The karyotype or chromosome count of your baby will reveal whether or not he has Translocation Trisomy 21.

The least common form of Down syndrome is known as Mosaicism. Only about 1 percent of all people with Down syndrome have this type of Trisomy 21. In Mosaicism, a faulty cell division occurs in one of the earliest cell divisions *after* fertilization. This is in contrast to other types of Down syndrome when the mistake in cell division occurs at or before fertilization. As in Nondisjunction Trisomy 21, something causes the chromosomes to divide unevenly. But when this occurs in the second or

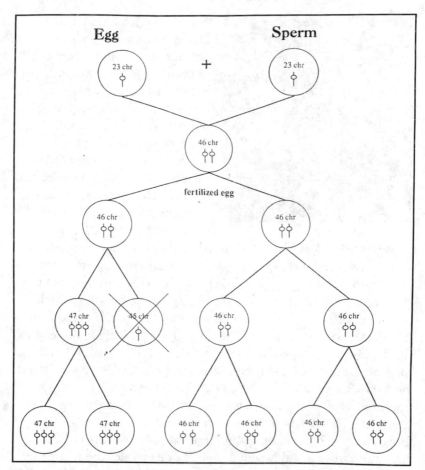

Figure 9: Mosaicism. A fertilized egg begins to divide normally. Nondisjunction occurs in one cell line resulting in an individual with both normal and trisomy cell lines.

third cell division, only some of the cells of the growing embryo contain the extra chromosome. As a result, not all the cells have the extra chromosome, and the baby may have fewer of the usual physical features as well as higher intellectual abilities. How the baby is affected depends not on the number of normal cells the baby has, but on where these cells are in the body. Figure 9 shows how Mosaicism occurs.

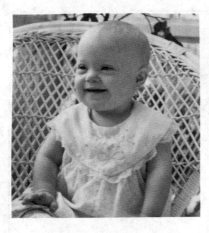

Although babies with Down syndrome possess an extra number-21 chromosome, all of their other chromosomes are normal. In fact, the material in the number-21 chromosomes is normal as well; there is just too much of it. Although the mechanism is still unknown, the additional chromosomal material, or trisomy, that results from the presence of three copies of the number-21 chromosome causes a genetic imbalance that alters the normal course of growth and development. Further, scientists have recently determined that only a portion of the number-21 chromosome contributes to Down syndrome. There appears to be a very small segment, or *critical region*, on chromosome 21 that, if present in triplicate, produces Down syndrome. This critical region resides in the lower part of chromosome 21. Figure 10 illustrates the part of the number-21 chromosome that causes Down syndrome and shows several of the genes that have been located on chromosome 21. Doctors and scientists speculate that these genes cause the Down syndrome features. In addition, scientists believe that the extra genetic material causes *incomplete* rather than abnormal growth and development. For example, the heart in people with Down syndrome is essentially normal, but the wall separating the two sides of the heart often is not completely developed. Similarly, the separation of the fingers is incomplete, resulting occasionally in webbed fingers.

In Down syndrome, only the number-21 chromosome pair is affected by the extra genetic material. The rest of your baby's chromosomes function normally, and that is why your baby seems so much like any other baby. Some of his features are affected by the extra number-21 chromosome, but most of his characteristics are determined by the remaining 46 chromosomes in his genetic blueprint.

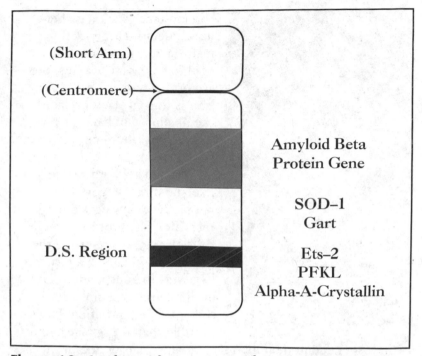

Figure 10: A schematic representation of chromosome 21 depicting the location of several genes and the Down Syndrome critical region. Every chromosome has a constriction called the centromere that divides it into a short and a long arm. The D.S. region is located on the long arm.

One of the many myths surrounding Down syndrome is that a child can have only "a little" Down syndrome. With the exception of Mosaicism, a child either has Down syndrome or does not. It is simply all in the genes.

Why Does My Child Have Down Syndrome?

Scientists have investigated the causes of Down syndrome for decades. So far its exact cause—what makes the number-21

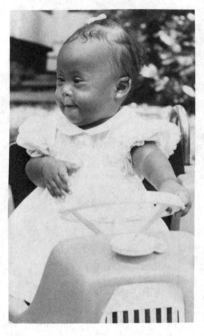

chromosomes stick together—has eluded discovery. Although many factors have been considered to be possible causes, the age of the mother (maternal age) is the only factor related to the likelihood of having a baby with Down syndrome that has been proven.

Women are born with a fixed number of eggs and do not produce new eggs during their life. The process of meiosis in the eggs starts while the woman is still herself a fetus. Eggs stay in a suspended state until meiosis is completed shortly before ovulation. It is possible that as eggs age and remain suspended in their meiosis for many years or decades, something happens to cause the chromosomes to become sticky or to fail to separate properly. Nondisjunction may also come from the father's sperm in about 10 to 15 percent of babies with Down syndrome. Even though a man produces new sperm throughout his adult life, scientists think that some men may be genetically predisposed to "sticky" genes. However, the hard fact remains that we don't know why Down syndrome occurs and we don't know how to prevent it. Research into the cause of Down syndrome continues.

Figure 11 shows the likelihood of having a baby with Down syndrome based on the mother's age at delivery. As you can see, the chance increases dramatically as women age. Yet many young women with no history of Down syndrome in their families have babies with Down syndrome. A surprising fact is that 75 percent of babies with Down syndrome are born to mothers under 35 years of age. This is because women under the age of 35 have far more babies than women over 35, and are less likely to have prenatal testing.

Figure 11. Likelihood of Having a Baby with Down Syndrome Based on Maternal Age

Maternal Age (Years)*	Estimated Risk	Maternal Age (Years)*	Estimated Risk
20	1/1231	35	1/274
21	1/1145	36	1/213
22	1/1065	37	1/166
23	1/1000	38	1/129
24	1/942	39	1/100
25	1/887	40	1/78
26	1/842	41	1/61
27	1/798	42	1/47
28	1/755	43	1/37
29	1/721	44	1/29
30	1/685	45	1/22
31	1/650	46	1/17
32	1/563	47	1/13
33	1/452	48	1/10
34	1/352	49	1/8

* This chart lists only the approximate frequency of babies with Down syndrome based on the mother's age at delivery. (Hook, E.B., Cross, P.K., and Schreinemachers, D.M. [1983] *JAMA* 249:2034)

What Are Babies with Down Syndrome Like?

Doctors are often able to spot babies with Down syndrome immediately after birth. Typically, newborns with Down syndrome have differences in their faces, neck, hands and feet, and muscle tone. The cluster of these features triggers the doctor's suspicions. After examining your baby, the doctor will usually order chromosome studies to confirm the diagnosis.

The following characteristics are most commonly associated with Down syndrome. Bear in mind, however, that there is tremendous variety among babies with Down syndrome; not every baby possesses all of the characteristic features. Most importantly, no connection has been shown between the number of Down syndrome features a baby has and that baby's cognitive ability.

Low Muscle Tone

Babies with Down syndrome have low muscle tone, called *hypotonia*. This means that their muscles appear relaxed and feel "floppy." Low tone usually affects all the muscles of the body. It is a significant physical feature that alerts doctors to look for other signs of Down syndrome. More importantly, low muscle tone affects your baby's movement, strength, and development. Most of the physical features linked to Down syndrome do not affect your baby's ability to grow and learn, but low muscle tone can complicate all areas of development. For example, low muscle tone affects the development of skills like rolling over, sitting, standing, and walking. Another area where low muscle tone can affect your baby's development is feeding and acceptance of solid food because the muscles in the mouth have low muscle tone.

Hypotonia cannot be cured. That is, your child's muscle tone will likely always be somewhat lower than other children's. Often, however, it can improve over time and can be improved by physical therapy. Accordingly, great importance is placed on good physical therapy to help children with low muscle tone develop properly, especially when they are very young. Physical therapy is discussed in Chapter 7.

Facial Features

Your baby's face may have some or all of the features characteristic of Down syndrome:

Nose. Your baby's face may be slightly broader and his nasal bridge may be flatter than usual. Often, children with Down syndrome have noses that are smaller than those of other children. The nasal passages may be smaller as well, and can become congested more quickly. Problems with nasal congestion are discussed in Chapter 3.

Eyes. Your child's eyes may appear to slant upward. This is why Down syndrome was formerly called "mongolism" because of the somewhat oriental appearance. Your doctor may call these *slant-*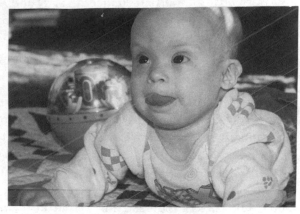*ing palpebral fissures.* The eyes may also have small folds of skin, called *epicanthal folds,* at the inner corners. The outer part of the iris (or colored part) of each eye may have light spots called *Brushfield spots.* These spots are more commonly seen in children with blue eyes. They do not affect your baby's sight and are not readily noticeable. It is very important to have your baby's eyesight checked, however, because vision problems tend to be more common in children with Down syndrome than in other children. This is discussed in more detail in Chapter 3.

Mouth. Your baby's mouth may be small, and the roof of his mouth may be shallow. When these features are accompanied by low muscle tone, the tongue may protrude or appear large in relation to the mouth.

Teeth. Your child's teeth may come in late and in an unusual order. Babies usually get their teeth in the same sequence, but the teeth of babies with Down syndrome seem to have a sequence all their own. The teeth may also be small, unusually shaped, and out of place, and these problems may continue when your child gets his permanent teeth.

Ears. Your baby's ears can be small and the tops may fold over. In addition, the ears of some babies with Down syndrome are set slightly lower on the head. The ear passages tend also to be smaller, which can make it very difficult for your pediatrician to check your baby's ears for infection. Because they are smaller, the ear passages can become blocked, causing a hearing loss. For this reason it is important to include early audiological exams in your infant's check-up schedule. Ear and hearing problems are discussed in Chapter 3.

Head Shape

Babies with Down syndrome have smaller than normal heads. Usually their head size falls within the lower 3 percent on standard growth charts for children. This is technically called *microcephaly*. The difference in size, however, is not usually noticeable. Studies have shown that the head, while smaller than average, is still within a normal range relative to the rest of the body. The back of the head may be flatter (*brachycephaly*). Also, the neck may appear shorter, and in newborns there may be loose folds of skin on the back of the neck, but these folds tend to disappear with growth. The soft spots of the head (*fontanels*), which are present in all babies, may be larger in babies with Down syndrome and may take longer to close in the normal course of development.

Stature

Babies with Down syndrome are usually of average weight and length at birth, but they do not grow as fast as do other children. For this reason, special growth charts for boys and girls with Down syndrome are used. During routine checkups, your doctor will measure your baby and plot the height and weight on the growth chart to make sure he is gaining weight nicely and growing well. Adolescents with Down syndrome achieve their final height around 15 years of age. The average adult height for males is 5 feet, 2 inches and in females 4½ feet. As discussed in Chapter 3, adolescents and adults with Down syndrome are prone to obesity.

Hands and Feet

Your child's hands may be smaller, and his fingers may be shorter, than other children's. The palm of each hand may have only one crease across it (a *transverse palmar or simian crease*), and the fifth finger may curve inward slightly with only one crease. Usually, the feet of babies with Down syndrome appear normal, but there may be a gap between the first and second toes. Frequently there is a deep crease on the sole of the feet in this gap.

Other Physical Features

Chest. Your baby's chest may be somewhat funnel shaped (when the chest bone is depressed) or pigeon breasted (bowing out of the chest wall). Neither of these differences in shape results in medical problems.

Skin. Your child's skin can be mottled, fair, and sensitive to irritation. Skin care is discussed in Chapter 4.

Hair. Children with Down syndrome typically have hair that is thin, soft, and often sparse.

Most newborns with Down syndrome do not exhibit all of the physical features described here. In general, the most common features are the low muscle tone, the upwardly slanting eyes, and the small ears. With the sole exception of low muscle tone, these features will not hinder either the health or the proper functioning of your baby. There are, however, some medical conditions associated with Down syndrome that can affect your baby's health. These are discussed in detail in Chapter 3.

Because your baby with Down syndrome has the extra chromosome, he may have features that resemble other babies with Down syndrome in some ways. However, because your baby also has twenty-two sets of completely normal chromosomes, he will also resemble his parents, brothers, and sisters, and will possess his own unique characteristics.

What About My Baby's Intelligence?

Babies with Down syndrome have mental retardation. That is, they learn more slowly and have difficulty with complex reasoning and judgment. The degree of mental retardation, however, varies tremendously. Your baby *will* learn; and what he learns, he will not "lose." Most importantly, remember that

Figure 12. Range of Human Intelligence

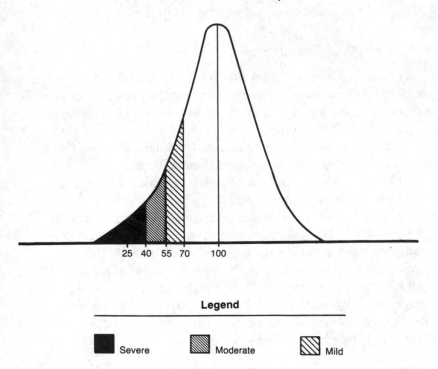

Distribution of IQ Scores in Population

25 40 55 70   100

Legend

Severe   Moderate   Mild

both the intellectual and the social skills of babies with Down syndrome are maximized when they are raised in a supportive environment with their families.

Intelligence has been measured for many years by standardized tests. Scores are often computed into a measurement called an *intelligence quotient* or *IQ*. This gauges a child's ability to reason, conceptualize, and think.

Among the general population, there is a wide range of measured intelligence (IQ). Studies find that ninety-five percent of the population have what is called "normal" intelligence, with IQs in the range of 70 to 130. Two and one-half percent of the population have what is called superior intelligence, with IQs over 130. And, two and one-half percent have intelligence below the normal range, with IQs of less than 70. Individuals who score below the normal range are considered to have mental retardation.

Just as there is a range for "normal" intelligence, there is also a range for mental retardation, called *degrees*. A person is considered to have mild mental retardation if his IQ range is between 55 and 70. Moderate mental retardation means an IQ range of between 40 and 55. Severe mental retardation means an IQ range of between 25 and 40. Figure 12 shows the full range of human intelligence on a bell curve. Most children with Down syndrome score within the moderate to mild range of mental retardation. Some children have more severe mental retardation, and some possess intelligence in the near-normal range.

Never forget that your child's IQ scores do not preclude him from taking care of himself, performing productive work, and, most importantly, learning. One of the myths that has long plagued children with Down syndrome is that because of their relatively lower IQ scores they cannot learn. This is simply not true.

Scientists do not yet understand how the extra chromosome in Down syndrome affects mental ability. Research indicates that the excess chromosome material in the number-21 chromosomes prevents or interferes with normal brain development. Both the size and structural complexity of the brain are different in babies with Down syndrome, but just how (or if) this affects mental functioning remains unknown. The human brain controls almost all of our bodies' functions, including muscle coordination, the five senses, intelligence, and behavior. Differences in chromosomes, such as Down syndrome, affect the brain and central nervous system, resulting in developmental delays or mental retardation.

Mental retardation has been misunderstood for centuries. As a result, society has consistently underestimated the intellectual potential of children with Down syndrome. Today, however, with appropriate treatment for medical conditions, early infant intervention, better education, and higher expectations, mental achievement for children with Down syndrome is on the

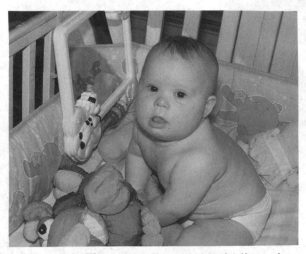

rise. Watch out for old studies and statistics about the mental ability of children with Down syndrome (usually gathered from people in institutions where there was no special education or early intervention). These studies tend to indicate lower intelligence than the more current studies show.

Children with Down syndrome have long suffered from low expectations and self-fulfilling negative prophecies. In the past, lower IQs condemned these children to institutions where, segregated from society, isolated, given little education, and quite often ignored, they could not surpass the low expectations held for them. Too often, low expectations yielded low performance. We know today that this negative cycle is both unfortunate *and* avoidable. With early infant intervention, advanced medical care, better education, and greater social acceptance, children with Down syndrome are functioning at increasingly higher levels. Not only are IQ scores on the rise, but new skills are learned and fuller lives are realized.

How will mental retardation affect your child? Although its effects are different in each child, mental retardation will generally slow development. Your child will learn new skills more slowly than other children, he will find it more difficult to pay attention for extended periods of time, his memory may not function as well as other children's, and he will have more trouble applying what he learns in one setting to another (called *generalization*). He will also find learning advanced skills harder. Skills requiring fast judgment, intricate coordination, and detailed analysis will be more difficult for him. This does not mean he can never develop advanced skills; but it will be harder and will take more time for him to learn these skills. The effect of mental retardation on your baby's development is discussed in Chapter 6.

Children with Down syndrome *can* learn. Parents often want to know precisely what skills their child will master. Will he be able to read? Will he learn to write? What will his schooling be like? None of these questions can be answered unequivocally for *any* child. Many children with Down syndrome learn to read and write. Many are included in regular classes throughout school. Remember that "normal" children also have a wide range of abilities, just as children with Down syndrome do.

There is much more to good development than reading and writing, and babies with Down syndrome do quite well with help. Although they may not excel in academic subjects or in complex reasoning, they can experience learning, achievement, and pride.

What About My Child's Future?

Generally speaking, children with Down syndrome can grow up to function with a great deal of independence. With the trend toward community living options, like group homes and apartments that foster independence and self-reliance, fewer and fewer adults with Down syndrome are remaining at home. They take care of themselves, hold jobs, and enjoy family and friends. As Chapter 8 explains, laws today protect all people with disabilities from the discrimination that formerly deprived them of so many opportunities. So, today there is real opportunity for learning, growth, and productivity throughout life. Achieving independence and self-reliance, however, takes a lot of effort. The essential foundation that will enable your child to grow into a capable adult is laid through hard work in the first years of life.

As children with Down syndrome grow up, parents often worry about their child's reproductive capacity. The concerns are different for male and female children. Men with Down syndrome cannot produce children, due either to a lack of or low sperm count or some other as-yet undiscovered reason. They do, however, grow and mature sexually. Most women with Down syndrome are fertile, but their eggs are likely to possess the extra number-21 chromosome. Consequently, it is likely that they will give birth to a baby with Down syndrome. Sex education and proper birth control methods are important subjects for you to discuss with your child as he or she grows.

Future Babies

Parents often wonder if their chances of having another baby with Down syndrome are higher after giving birth to a child with Down syndrome. The answer depends both on the type of Down syndrome your child has and on your particular family history.

In general, the risk of having another baby with Down syndrome is one in one hundred, *regardless of the mother's age,* unless the woman is already over 40. This represents a large increase in risk for mothers who are under thirty. As Figure 11 shows, the risk in the general population does not approach one in one hundred until approximately age 39. After 39, the probability increases markedly. These figures apply to families with a child with Nondisjunction Trisomy 21, or roughly 95 percent of all families with a child with Down syndrome.

For families who have a baby with Translocation Down syndrome, the risk of recurrence is also about one in one hundred unless the condition is inherited from either parent. When it is inherited from a parent, the risk of recurrence is significantly higher than in the general population. In this case, the risk of recurrence depends on the type of translocation and the sex of the carrier parent. If the mother is the carrier, the risk is about one in ten; if the father is the carrier, the risk is about one in twenty. To find out exactly what type of Down syndrome your baby has, ask your geneticist. He or she can tell from looking at your baby's karyotype and will counsel you accordingly. If necessary, your chromosomes can be tested to determine whether or not you carry a balanced translocation.

Prenatal Tests to Detect Down Syndrome

Following the birth of a baby with Down syndrome, or if your doctor determines that you are at increased risk of giving birth to a baby with Down syndrome, you can monitor future pregnancies with either *amniocentesis* or *chorionic villi sampling (CVS)*. These common prenatal tests are used to determine a fetus's chromosomes during pregnancy. Amniocentesis is typically performed around the sixteenth week of pregnancy, either in a doctor's office or in a hospital. Before the procedure, the doctor performs an ultrasound scan which shows the location of the uterus, placenta, amniotic fluid, and fetus. During the procedure, a very thin needle is inserted into the uterus through the mother's abdomen. A small amount of amniotic fluid is drawn out and analyzed. Because the amniotic fluid contains cells from the fetus, doctors are able to thoroughly examine the cells and count the chromosomes to determine whether the baby has Down syndrome or any other chromosome disorder. It generally takes about twelve to fourteen days to obtain results.

Since its introduction in the late 1960s, amniocentesis has been performed during hundreds of thousand of pregnancies. Although amniocentesis is a very safe procedure and is almost considered to be routine, a small percentage of complications have been reported. These include miscarriages (less than 1 in 200), cramping, and bleeding.

Chorionic villus sampling (CVS) is a newer prenatal procedure that is done early in pregnancy between nine and eleven weeks of gestation. CVS is no longer an experimental procedure and is considered to be safe and accurate when it is done by an experienced physician and the tissue is analyzed by a laboratory with expertise in handling the sample. Following an ultrasound, a thin tube is inserted through the vagina and a small piece of *chorionic villi*, the projections of tissue from the placenta, is obtained. Sometimes, depending on the woman's anatomy or the location of the fetus, the tissue may be obtained by inserting a thin needle through the abdomen. Because cells from the villi are fetal tissue, they can be cultured for their chromosome content in one week to ten days. In terms of side effects, CVS is slightly more likely than amniocentesis to be followed by miscarriage or other complications such as infection, bleeding, and leaking of amniotic fluid from the vagina.

Which particular diagnostic test to use—CVS or amniocentesis—depends on personal preference, the available expertise in your area, and your medical history. Your doctor should be able to guide you to the appropriate procedure.

Prenatal Blood Tests to Detect Down Syndrome

In the past few years, scientists and doctors have introduced new blood tests to detect Down syndrome during pregnancy. *Alpha-feto protein (AFP)* is a protein produced by all fetuses during pregnancy. This protein is found in the baby's blood, the mother's blood, and the amniotic fluid. A low level of AFP in the mother's blood can indicate the possible presence of Down syndrome. It is thus called a *marker*.

More recently, tests for other markers have been developed. Combined screening for multiple markers is referred to as *triple screen* or *triple test*, and is rapidly becoming a common practice. The triple test, like alpha-feto protein testing, is a blood test that is offered to pregnant women between the 15th and 20th week of gestation. *Triple test is not a diagnostic test.* It is only a screening test designed to look for potential problems and to calculate the probability of having a baby with a genetic defect. Currently, triple tests can detect fetuses with Down syndrome 60 percent of the time.

If abnormal levels are found, you should be referred for an ultrasound examination or a sonogram that may detect the cause of the abnormal levels. These causes may include inaccurate estimate of length of gestation, or the presence of twins, as well as a variety of other birth defects. Amniocentesis is frequently recommended to confirm a diagnosis.

Although advanced tests may permit you to learn the chromosomal make-up of your future babies, this knowledge can create a dilemma. If tests show Down syndrome, you may have to make some painful and difficult decisions. Of course, the most intimate personal decisions are involved, and this book does not presume to recommend to you what to do about future pregnancies.

The History of Down Syndrome

Well before the genetic link to Down syndrome was discovered, John Langdon Down, an English physician, described the condition as a distinct set of characteristics. In 1866, he distinguished Down syndrome from other conditions by noting some of the common features associated with it, such as straight, thin hair, a small nose, and a broad face. Down is also responsible for naming the condition "mongolism." Through the years, terms like "mongoloid idiot" have been used. These and other derogatory labels are no longer commonly used today, though people still need to be reminded that Down syndrome does not refer to someone who is unhappy or inferior. It seems that too few people realize that Down syndrome is named for the man credited with first describing it.

In this century, advances in genetic research helped scientists begin to understand the cause of Down syndrome. By the early 1930s, some researchers began to suspect that Down syndrome might be caused by a chromosomal abnormality. In 1959, Jerome Lejune, a French geneticist, discovered that cells grown from individuals with Down syndrome had an extra chromosome. Later, the exact location of the extra chromosome was found to be at the number-21 chromosome. These findings led to the discovery of the other forms of Down syndrome, including Translocation and Mosaicism.

The treatment of people with Down syndrome has also advanced remarkably over the decades. Life spans have increased dramatically with improved medical care, and the education and care of people with Down syndrome have also improved markedly. For years children with Down syndrome were thought to have no potential to learn. Denied the opportunity to learn, they seemed to confirm society's mistakenly low estimation of their abilities. Thankfully, today's world is very different for children with Down syndrome.

Recent Progress in Down Syndrome

Doctors, scientists, and researchers continue to explore the causes, effects, and treatment of Down syndrome. With technological advances in the field of modern genetics, scientists are isolating individual genes and studying their specific functions. Researchers are also probing to discover just how the extra chromosome causes the characteristics of Down syndrome and why some people with Down syndrome have certain features (such as heart defects) and others do not. Scientists have already identified many of the thousands of genes on the twenty-first chromosome. Their goal is to pinpoint the genes that cause Down syndrome, and then "decode" their biochemical processes.

Over time, much will be learned about Down syndrome. Some doctors are working on ways to alter the appearance of children with Down syndrome to reduce some of the features associated with it, such as the slanting eyes and protruding tongue, in order to lessen the stigma that has often accompanied the condition. Though controversial and unproven, if this interests you, consult your child's pediatrician or geneticist. Generally speaking, plastic surgery is not performed on infants

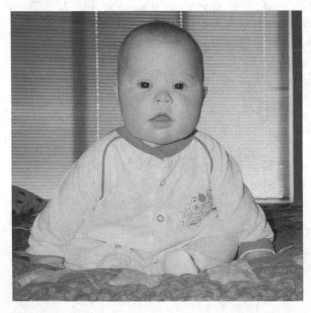

or very young children. Your specialists can keep you informed of the most current treatments in this area.

Parents need to be wary, however. Often parents and doctors hear of "cures" for Down syndrome. People have claimed that megavitamins (huge doses of vitamins), enzymes, sicca cells, amino acids, and experimental drugs can reduce the degree of mental retardation. None of the claims has yet proved true. Some experimental treatments can even be dangerous to your child.

It is possible that some of the ongoing research in these areas may yield solid results in the future, but so far no treatment or cure has been found. Although there is room for experimental, creative treatments designed to help children with Down syndrome reach their potential, false claims and empty promises only hurt families.

Conclusion

It is vital that you learn as much as you can about Down syndrome. Many books about Down syndrome, mental retardation, and children with disabilities are available. But be careful: *avoid books that are outdated*. The Reading List at the end of this book contains a list of useful current sources. In addition, many of the organizations listed in the Resource Guide in the back of this book can also direct you to useful materials.

Down syndrome has its own language. Understanding the terms used in connection with your child's care and development is important for good communication with doctors, teachers, and other professionals. The glossary at the end of this book will help. You will be surprised by how fast you will become an "expert" in Down syndrome and by how much a good understanding of Down syndrome will help you and your child.

REFERENCES

Cheng, E.Y., Luthy, D.A., Zeblman, A.M., Williams, M.A., Lieppman R.E., Hickok D.E. "A Prospective Evaluation of a Second-Trimester Screening Test for Fetal Down Syndrome using Maternal Serum Alpha-Fetoprotein, hCG, and Unconjugated Estriol." *Obstetrics & Gynecology.* Vol. 81, 1993, 72–77.

Canick, J.A., Knight, G.J. "Multiple-Marker Screening for Fetal Down Syndrome." *Contemporary OB/GYN.* April, 1992, 3–12.

Korenberg, J.R., Kawashima, H., Pulst, S.M., Ikeuchi, T., Ogasawara, N., Yamamoto, K., Schonber, S.A., West, R., Allen, L., Magenis, E., Ikawa, K., Taniguche, N., Epstein, C.J. "Molecular Definition of a Region of

Chromosome 21 That Causes Features of the Down Syndrome Pheno-
type." *American Journal of Human Genetics.* Vol. 47, 1990, 236–246.
Serra, A., Neri, G. "Trisomy 21: Conference Report and 1990 Update."
Am.J.Med.Genet. Vol. 7, 1990, 11–19.

Parent Statements

I remember my image of Down syndrome before Michael was
born—the Psych. 101 films of insane asylums and state institutions, bleak, black-and-white films. The reality is radically different.

I'd never known a child with Down syndrome. I had worked a
little with adults with Down syndrome, and it was horrible.
They were very poorly functioning individuals. No speech, minimal comprehension of receptive speech or language, just very
low functioning. But those people were institutionalized since
birth. Whereas my husband knew a family who raised their
daughter with Down syndrome at home and he has followed her
progress for many years. She is now about fourteen and does
very well. Also, we had good information. We had a geneticist
who knew what could happen, that a child could function very
well or very poorly, and explained the need for early intervention right from the beginning. I think we need more health professionals who are educated to push parents in this direction.

We were real surprised to find out how common Down syndrome is. We thought it was just women over 40 who gave birth
to babies with Down syndrome.

When Josh was born, we were surprised at how common Down
syndrome was. And not only Down syndrome, but mental retardation in general. We wanted to pick up a lot of information. Of

course the biggest question is the one they can't answer: "What's causing this? How does Down syndrome make him the way he is?"

~ ~ ~ ~ ~ ~ ~ ~ ~

We had even talked about adopting a child with Down syndrome. That was probably a year and a half before Julie was born. I think we thought about it so hard we split a chromosome.

~ ~ ~ ~ ~ ~ ~ ~ ~

My image of what Down syndrome was before our son was born was not very clear. I don't think I knew the connection between the word "mongoloid" and "Down syndrome." I remember there was a boy with Down syndrome who lived in our neighborhood before Christopher was born, and he perplexed me because he seemed able to get about by himself, but he looked like he had mental retardation at the same time.

~ ~ ~ ~ ~ ~ ~ ~ ~

I had a fear of having a child with a disability, and when our child was born with Down syndrome, I was scared. Mental retardation or mental problems were very foreign and strange to me.

~ ~ ~ ~ ~ ~ ~ ~ ~

I knew the incidence of Down syndrome was about one in six hundred. That meant it wouldn't happen to me, right? Now I tend to think that things will go wrong. I mean, when someone says to me, one in six hundred, it's like saying, "Well, there's a great possibility that it will happen."

~ ~ ~ ~ ~ ~ ~ ~ ~

It took me five years and tens of thousands of dollars in infertility treatments to get pregnant. So, even though I was 36 and knew I had an increased risk of having a baby with Down syndrome, I didn't have an amnio. I figured that, statistically, I was much more likely to have a miscarriage as the result of the amnio than I was to have a baby with Down syndrome. So much for playing the odds! The second time around, I didn't care about the risks of prenatal testing. The reason I wanted to have a second child was so my first child would have a "normal" sibling to help her out after my husband and I died. So, I had CVS at ten weeks gestation. The baby didn't have Down syndrome and I didn't have a miscarriage. I'm still not sure what we would have done if our second baby had turned out to have Down syndrome, too.

If I had any impression about Down syndrome when my son was born, it was that he'd just be a blob and he would never walk or talk and he'd just be a total vegetable. But then I found out that's not true. He has a very definite personality.

I haven't really worked with kids with Down syndrome but I've seen lots of them. I was working in special ed centers but with older children. None of the kids I worked with had Down syndrome. But I just loved the kids with Down syndrome. I liked being with them and I liked their vivaciousness and just lots of things about them.

After Chris was born, we wanted to learn. All we had to go on was half of a column of a page about Down syndrome in a medical book. The book said that these children are quite sociable and if possible, parents should try and bring them up at home, they make wonderful pets. You know, it didn't say that, but could have. We were really thirsting for knowledge.

I know a lot of women who are well into their thirties. One of them was pregnant and close to forty. She was having her first baby, and was having amniocentesis. She came and asked me for counsel, and flat out said she would probably abort if she found out the baby had Down syndrome. I don't like to get into the abortion issue, but I was just real candid on the fact that Julie is the joy of our lives. She's brought such an added dimension to our lives. In a lot of ways she's difficult, but it's a different type of workload. But boy, she's not a liability; she's a definite asset.

It was a struggle to get good information. We were lucky because I was in the special ed business. I had friends who had friends who immediately could refer me to parents or doctors or books. I think that a lot of parents have to seek those out and don't know where to go to get them.

My child has something called "partial trisomy 21." Her extra chromosome 21 is missing a little piece. Nobody, including the geneticist, can tell us much about what to expect. We do know that how she is affected depends on which Down syndrome characteristics are usually caused by the missing piece. In the beginning, we worried a lot about how she would be affected. She's doing great now, however.

I can't imagine putting a child in an institution. When I look at my little boy and see how he takes my existence so absolutely for granted, it's impossible to imagine my not being there for him. It's not so much that he's mine, but that I'm his. He has no concept of belonging to me less than his sister just because he has Down syndrome.

I keep putting Julie into a historical perspective of generations who were sent off to institutions or who were kept in the closet. They were lumps on logs—you kept them clean and that was about it. And now, we're moving into an era where the whole generation is being mainstreamed. Even if we stopped doing anything special for Julie, just the fact that she's in a family where she's accepted, she's light years ahead.

You learn day by day. I imagine we'll always be learning. There's something new around every corner about her and about how society reacts to her. It's a constant learning process. And you have to educate doctors, friends, and neighbors. We're still kind of new in this neighborhood. A lot of the neighbors are real interested, and that's nice, but it's a constant education process.

Two

～～～～～

Adjusting To
Your New Baby

Marilyn Trainer*

Getting the News

It is painful beyond belief to be told that your precious new baby has Down syndrome. Instead of feeling that special sense of joy, all those months of waiting end with your world turned upside down. During those months you didn't care whether it would be a girl or a boy—you just wanted a healthy baby. But the baby you were expecting never arrived.

Your baby has Down syndrome. And you have another kind of syndrome: "Why us?" It is a syndrome that strikes virtually every family who has had a child with mental retardation. It's almost as if a stark, impenetrable wall has dropped from somewhere and with terrible force cut off the future, not only for the small new baby, whom none of you yet really know, but for all of you in ways you cannot explain, but instinctively know are there.

You are in shock. In the minute or so after you first hear the term "Down syndrome," a strange, almost warm feeling envelops you. You are sitting inside a bubble; you can hear voices, and

---

*   Marilyn Trainer is the parent of a young adult with Down syndrome. She has been active for many years with The Arc and Parents of Down Syndrome Children. She is the author of *Differences in Common: Straight Talk on Down Syndrome, Mental Retardation, and Life* (Woodbine House 1991). Her writing has appeared in the *Washington Post* and other publications.

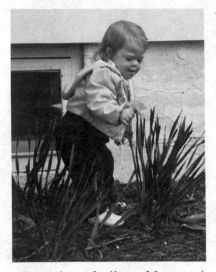

you can respond to them. But somebody else is sitting in that bubble. The real you is outside, far above, watching and listening. You feel calm, except that you're trembling from head to toe. If you could just stay there above the bubble, if you could just stay there safe and untouched—but of course you can't. And so reality begins.

This chapter addresses what the reality of having a baby with Down syndrome feels like and what you can do about those feelings. No one should tell you how to feel right now: there is no preprogrammed response to being told your baby has Down syndrome. Soon you will begin to notice all the little things that are just like any other baby—soft warm skin, tiny fingers and toes, cries for Mom or Dad—and your need to care for your baby will take over.

Your Emotions

All kinds of emotions well up at once: anger, despair, guilt, shame, rejection—yes, rejection of the baby—and perhaps most of all, a terrible fear of the future. You wonder how you are going to cope with this overwhelming burden for the rest of your lives.

Will life ever be even remotely light and carefree again? Will there always be a feeling of never-ending responsibility with no light at the end of the tunnel? Will there ever be laughter again or has the funny side of life been lost forever along with happiness? Many parents in the days following the birth of a child with disabilities are plagued by these and other fears.

Grief

Often the first reaction to the news that your baby has Down syndrome is intense grief and sorrow. You may grieve the loss of that ideal baby you dreamed of or the loss of your family's "normalcy." You may not even know exactly why you are grieving. What you do know, however, is that sorrow sits on your chest like a ton of bricks. This sense of grief is, for parents who have received such shocking news, completely normal. And as with most parents, your grief will pass eventually.

But right now you may be feeling as if your heart will surely break. How could this have happened? How could this have happened to *you?* The unfairness of it is beyond comprehension. Worse, how will you face up to years of a responsibility that seems so totally overwhelming and one which you fear you cannot possibly handle? You lie awake at night consumed with worry and if you do fall asleep your dreams are so disturbing that you awake in panic. Are dreams any worse than the reality, your tired mind may ask?

It's easy to let your grief rob you of the joyful feelings you can experience at your baby's birth. You went through all those months of pregnancy; you delivered your baby. You *have* achieved the miracle of life—your baby, alive, loving, and entirely trusting in you. Your love for your baby will grow spontaneously and will conquer the grief.

Ego

Ego can be the biggest obstacle to accepting your child. Its interference is perfectly normal, and, as with other negative feelings, will diminish over time.

There is no denying that for many parents the birth of a child with disabilities is a tremendous blow to self-esteem. How could *we* produce a child with screwed-up chromosomes, they ask? *Other* people have children with disabilities, we don't. It is simply not in *our* life plan. Along life's way it may be that some of our own goals will not be met, but one thing is for sure: Our children will be bright and beautiful and excel in all they do. When our children make it, we make it too.

Give your baby a chance. Your love will grow naturally and you will realize that your baby has great potential. Children with Down syndrome work so hard to achieve. Rather than feeling a blow to your ego, you will feel tremendous pride at what your child accomplishes.

Resentment and Depression

Parents usually experience other painful emotions that they would consider less than noble. Jealousy, resentment, depression, and rejection are all common emotions in people who receive shocking news. You may resent parents with "normal" babies, begrudging them the joy you know they feel. You even resent that they appear to take their baby's normalcy so much for granted. It can be especially difficult when others seem to treat the birth of your own baby as a death. Instead of flowers sent to your room in the hospital, you get silence or sympathy— no congratulatory cards or baby presents.

You wish you could feel joy over the birth of your baby but the pain is too strong. You may even wish your baby would die— that you could wake up freed from this nightmare. These feelings may strike you as contemptible. They are not; rather, they are your mind's way of coping with a situation you cannot fully grasp or control. Time and love will heal your wounds.

Anger

It is not unusual for some parents to feel a powerful anger and bitterness. Rarely is this directed toward the baby. Rather, it is a lashing out at fate, circumstances, even God. "How could God do this to us when we've tried so hard to live by his commandments?" This sense of betrayal is no small anguish. But as time passes and parents allow themselves to learn about Down syndrome, they realize that raging against the supernatural is about as productive as raging against the extra chromosome which is the true cause of Down syndrome.

You may not like feeling angry and bitter, but in admitting these feelings you are being honest and realistic. And it is important to be realistic. In the long run, your baby will be better for it. Consider the parents—and sadly there are some—who either refuse to believe the diagnosis or who believe God will work a miracle and "take the Down syndrome away from *our* baby." There are parents who refuse in any way to enhance opportunities for their baby's development; no infant stimulation, no early intervention, no participating in parents' groups, no learning about Down syndrome—no consideration of the baby's future as a child with special needs because God will "cure" it. Months, even years, pass; the parents wait for the miracle and the child loses precious ground which can never be made up. Please note; Down syndrome of itself is not a tragedy, but there are those who can make it so.

Go ahead, be angry. But don't let that anger debilitate you and don't sit around waiting for miracles either. Create your own miracles by converting your anger into energy, and use that energy to seek out and utilize every opportunity that comes your child's way. It's amazing what "angry" parents can accomplish when that anger is properly channeled.

Helplessness

To say that nobody gets through life without problems is as worn out a cliché as you can hear, even if it happens to be true. Many a parent has stated that until the day they had a child born with Down syndrome there wasn't any problem that they hadn't been able to solve. Whether they avoided the problem, dispensed with it themselves, or waited until it was resolved over time, the problem eventually went away. Down syndrome does not go away. When parents start thinking about this they are often overwhelmed by a sense of helplessness and vulnerability. "How can we ever make it right?" "How can we fix it?" Obviously, nobody's going to "fix" it. But take heart, for as you read through this book you will find that where your baby is concerned you will become anything but helpless. It may not seem possible now, but in a short while, you will become knowledgeable and active.

How to Adjust

Address Your Emotions

Right now you may understand the term "emotional roller coaster" as you never have before in your life. It probably never crossed your mind that you would be riding this particular roller coaster but here you are, like it or not. You are bringing a baby home feeling more than the usual newborn baby stress. The house is a mess, work responsibilities have fallen by the way, your other children need attention: there is always too much to do. Don't let the press of work prevent you from sifting your thoughts and emotions. Time spent on yourself now is essential.

Take Time to Adjust

You know best what you need to do first. Some people need to organize their lives. Others deal with their problems by jumping in head first. Still others need to be alone and withdrawn. Above all, take the time you need to adjust and recover. Don't make irreversible decisions immediately. You can't solve all the problems for your baby's life or your life right away.

Don't Feel Personally Responsible

Do you torture yourself in the belief that you have somehow "given" your child Down syndrome? We have all heard of babies who are born with problems because of things mothers did or did not do during pregnancy. We've all read how drugs, alcohol, tobacco, poor nutrition, or lack of prenatal care can affect a baby. Self-indulgence, ignorance, or plain stupidity can take a terrible toll. But the chromosomal abnormality of Down syndrome is not caused by any of these. You are not personally responsible for your baby's extra chromosome any more than you are responsible for the last raindrops to fall in your neighborhood.

Underneath the feeling of personal responsibility is that old feeling of guilt that you are somehow at fault for producing a damaged baby. And below that are feelings of guilt for rejecting this baby while longing for the baby that never was. It hurts even more when we see or hear of a mother who didn't do everything "right" during her pregnancy. Maybe she smoked, drank too much coffee or too many glasses of wine, or worse. Her baby turned out perfectly fine anyway. Your baby should have been born as fully endowed as any other baby. But fate or nature—call it what you will—cheated her, and in doing so cheated you too.

Quirks of fate or nature happen every day—often in worse ways than conceiving a baby with Down syndrome. You are no more responsible for your baby's Down syndrome than other parents are for their child's leukemia. So relinquish that guilt and put your energies where they are needed: in getting your strength back and helping your baby to reach her full potential.

Allow Yourself to Grieve

Right now all you may want to do is cry. Spill all the tears you want; you have the right. Rant and rave if that is your way; you have the right to that too. Or go somewhere to lick your wounds alone.

Whatever you do, there is something you should keep in mind: Hardly a parent of a child with Down syndrome has not experienced these very emotions with wrenching anguish. And although you may find it impossible to believe right now, almost every one of those parents would tell you that despite the initial heartache they would choose to have their child again a thousand times over. It's almost a sure bet that in not too many months you will be saying the same thing.

Sometimes old truths do well by us: Let some time pass. You *will* laugh again; your baby will see to that.

What You Should Do

Get to Know Your Baby

This might sound utterly banal considering what you are experiencing now, but ask yourself whether you are thinking more about the baby or more about the baby's condition. When you look at your baby do you see your child or do you see Down syndrome? Take your cue from a youngster with Down syndrome who when told he was "a living doll" replied indignantly, "I'm not a doll—I'm a person!" He's right; that baby of yours is a person and as you come to *know* that little person you will feel less grief. As you take on the pivotal role of helping your baby to develop, wounded pride and bruised ego become irrelevant. As a matter of fact, expanded horizons often bring a mature kind of pride: pride in what your baby is achieving and pride in the part you play.

Tell Your Friends and Family

There is no doubt that one of your most difficult tasks is to break the news about the baby to friends and relatives, particularly grandparents. Unfortunately, there are still those who are steeped in ignorance and prejudice. They may have grown up at a time when mental retardation was considered in the most negative way. They feel hurt just as you do, but may cast about for someone to blame, saying, "There's never been anything like this in the family before."

Sometimes grandparents can be particularly trying. For example, it's not unheard of for grandparents to pressure parents to place the child in an institution or up for adoption. When this

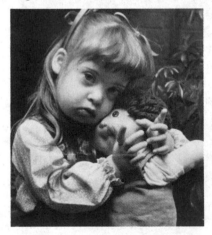

doesn't work, they may ignore the child as much as possible, never mentioning the baby to friends, much less bragging about the baby as grandparents are wont to do. This attitude can be devastating to parents who are in a very vulnerable state themselves and are struggling to cope and to accept their child.

Give grandparents, aunts, uncles, brothers, sisters, and

friends time to overcome their shock. Just as you needed some time to process the unexpected information, they need time to adjust as well. Their first reaction may not be their last.

Happily, people with negative attitudes about Down syndrome are in the minority. You must catch your breath, get your facts straight, and explain the situation in due time as forthrightly as possible. Give these people a book or pamphlet to read that presents an accurate picture of Down syndrome. They may know absolutely nothing about Down syndrome and may suffer from a distorted picture. Moreover, people will take their cue from you and most will become sincerely interested and involved with you and your baby. A good number of advocates for children with Down syndrome are friends and relatives who have no children with special needs of their own.

Some people may never "come around"; they may always suffer from old myths and stereotypes, excess pity, or other emotions. These people cannot matter—you have more important things to do, more important people to care for. Seek out people who will help *you* cope.

Contact Other Parents

One of the very best sources of support is other parents of children with Down syndrome. Down syndrome parent groups can be found in all parts of the country and throughout the world. You can even reach them via computer. Parents in the same boat can be tremendously helpful. Seek out an acquaintance, a small group, or an organization when you feel ready.

There are many ways to make contact. Try calling your local chapter of The Arc (formerly called the Association for Retarded Citizens), your local chapter of the March of Dimes, your local Down syndrome parents' group, or your school system. Ask to speak with a staff member who works with parents of children with disabilities. These and other groups who can help are noted in the Resource Guide at the end of this book.

If you feel put off by the idea of suddenly becoming involved with an organization, be assured that parent-to-parent groups are usually small and informal, and no one is going to try

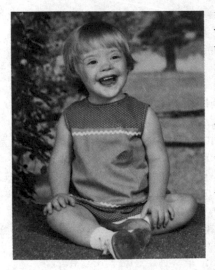

to "recruit you." Tell them you need someone to talk to who can give you some basic information. Your greatest support will almost always come from other parents. No one is going to understand you better. It's just a phone call; you have nothing to lose, and potentially a great deal to gain. Aside from support and valuable information, many parents develop lifelong friendships with other parents because their children happen to have an extra chromosome in common.

Round Up Your Professionals

Get as much help for your baby as you can. When you have a baby without special needs, you're often on your own. But when your baby does have special needs, you will be surprised at the number of experts out there who can help you. In fact, some parents, after benefitting from the phalanx of professionals lined up to help their baby, say that they could have used a little of this help for their "normal" children.

Throughout the book we describe the different kinds of people who can help your baby, along with what they do. They include educators, therapists, and a wide variety of doctors. There are pediatricians, cardiologists, internists, geneticists, ear, nose and throat specialists, and ophthalmologists. Each plays a key role in screening your baby for possible problems and in helping ensure that your child stays healthy.

You may find it helpful to use one doctor to coordinate the medical services your child might need. A pediatric geneticist who specializes in Down syndrome and other chromosomal conditions can be very helpful as a coordinator and information source. Ask your pediatrician, hospital, or obstetrician to refer you and your child.

Be prepared in case a doctor expresses outdated negative and inaccurate information. Unbelievably enough, there are a few who still recommend institutionalization or inaction or who express horribly negative outlooks. If your doctor is negative, change doctors. Parents are sometimes frustrated in trying to find a doctor who cares, but good doctors are out there. The search is worth the effort. Other parents are your best source of references to doctors who are good with kids and families with Down syndrome. Shop around, be picky, and get what is best for your child.

Keep Your Baby Home

Experienced parents will give new parents one essential message: *keep your baby home!* Resist pressure from anyone to do otherwise no matter who is doing the pressuring. Even if you are inclined to send your baby away, *don't do it!* There is absolutely no reason not to raise your child at home. You are in the best position to raise your child, to help her grow, to protect her rights. There are people out there to help you. Don't throw away the chance for a very fulfilling family experience, not to mention a lot of love.

For those relatively few parents who know in their heart of hearts that they will never be able to accept their baby as she deserves to be accepted, adoption is a viable reality. Did you know that there is a waiting list of over one hundred prospective parents who *want* to adopt babies with Down syndrome? The National Down Syndrome Congress has information about adoption, as does Chapter 5 of this book.

Get the Facts

Ignorance is your worst enemy. Don't let outdated assumptions about what the future holds for children with Down syndrome get the better of you. The prognosis for your child is much more positive than it would have been just ten to twenty years ago. In part this is due to advances in medical care, but it's also because the people who work with these kids know a great deal more about achieving the best possible developmental path for your child. One of the first priorities is to get some information. Read books, consult professionals, and talk to parents. Consult the Reading List at the back of this book.

But be careful what you read. Although information about Down syndrome has improved within the past ten years, there is still much antiquated material on library shelves. Some of this old information is enough to scare the wits out of new parents. Instead of visiting the public library, check with your local office of The Arc or one of the Down syndrome organizations to find out about reading matter. And don't forget that these groups are very good about mailing brochures, packets, and information to people in rural areas. Sometimes a small fee is required, but it is well worth the cost.

Teach Your Baby Now

The importance of early intervention cannot be stressed enough. Neither can the fact that you can motivate your child better than anyone. Early intervention means parents and professionals beginning work with a child when she is still a baby to help her reach her greatest potential. The normal developmental sequence of children is used as a guide. It's not just a matter of encouraging your baby to keep trying new and "harder" things, but to do them right. Early intervention requires professional help, but much of it can be done right at home. Under the law, your baby has a *right* to receive free early intervention services, beginning at birth. Chapters 6 and 7 address some of the fundamentals of development and how important early intervention is for your baby. Chapter 8 explains your child's rights to early intervention and special education. At home, and with professional help, you can truly enhance your baby's potential.

The goal of early intervention is to devise ways to increase your baby's learning abilities every chance you get. There are opportunities everywhere in your baby's daily life, if you think about it. For example, a cat or a dog can be a great incentive for

a child to move, or just to actively observe. Think about
the family who gives tender,
loving care to their ancient dia-
betic cat because years ago as
a frisky kitten she enticed a
baby to follow her—to roll, to
hitch, to crawl, and to walk.
(Today guess who most often
feeds her and holds her and
loves her?)

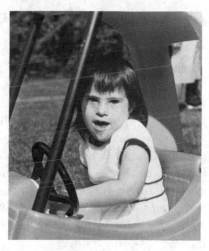

Your brand new baby obvi-
ously is not going to be chas-
ing the family cat. But a new
baby can do exercises that strengthen muscles and improve
tone, and can be introduced to playing games. Just remember
that early intervention is crucial in the development of a child
with Down syndrome and it should begin as soon as possible.
But don't get nervous; work with professionals, use your common sense, and try to have fun with it.

Don't Despair

Above all, the experienced parent will want to tell you, "Do
not despair." Don't even think of those things your child might
not be able to do. At this point there is almost nothing you can
rule out of your baby's future repertoire. Focus on what your
child can and will do *now*—all the better to help her seemingly
small achievements build toward future milestones.

It is important to keep your perspective and sense of hu-
mor. Minimize stress by having fun when you can. Get yourself
a babysitter—a close friend might really enjoy the opportunity—
and go out to dinner, a movie, whatever—regularly. A baby is a
baby after all, and there's no reason yours won't be just fine
with a reliable sitter. Babysitting is discussed more fully in
Chapter 4.

What About My Family?

Many parents ask whether a baby with Down syndrome will affect their other children. Chapter 5 addresses that question in detail, but a quick and easy answer is a resounding yes. Siblings of babies with Down syndrome will most certainly be affected.

One mother recalls the day she and her husband brought their baby home from the hospital. With sadness and great apprehension in her heart she wondered what this was going to mean to the lives of their three older children, a boy of ten and two girls, eight and four. The baby was placed in his bassinet in the parents' bedroom as the children gathered around to see their new baby brother. The baby needed changing so the mother removed the wet diaper. Before she could put on the fresh one, the baby urinated in a beautiful streaming arc that hit the wall and trickled down. The children's eyes widened in undisguised admiration. "Wow! Look what he can do!"

Overcome by a tremendous sense of relief, the mother didn't know whether to laugh or cry. It didn't matter in the least to those children that their baby brother had Down syndrome. In their eyes he had performed a fantastic feat and was a wonder of a baby. They loved him and that was that.

Many years have passed since that significant day, but no member of the family has ever forgotten it. Today that baby is a capable, high-functioning young adult, thanks in large part to his brother and sisters who with each goal he achieved said, "Wow! Look what he can do."

Certainly the lives of your other children will be changed now and in the future because their sibling has Down syndrome. No one in life is immune to change, but children adjust to it surprisingly well. It becomes a natural part of their world. There may be times when they are annoyed, bothered, or even embarrassed by their sibling with Down syndrome, but with good communication, understanding, and a lifetime of shared experiences, the deepest bonds will form. Chapter 5 discusses in detail the relationship of your baby with Down syndrome and her siblings.

And it is no coincidence that many brothers and sisters who have siblings with Down syndrome grow up to be unreservedly compassionate and understanding human beings. Even during those tumultuous teenage years youngsters who love and live with someone who has a disability exhibit insights about life—what is truly important, what is not—which their peers often sorely lack.

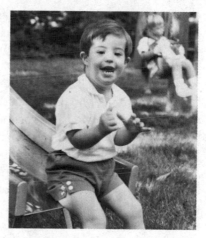

Almost every adult brother and sister will tell you that their sibling with Down syndrome has enriched their lives beyond all measure and they wouldn't trade her for the brightest, most beautiful child on the face of this Earth.

Your Work Will Pay Off

Kids with Down syndrome can do just about anything any other child can do. It might take them a little longer, but they can do it. They can learn to read, write, and use computers, and some parents report a positive genius in their children for reading logos and road signs that will take them to McDonald's or Pizza Hut. And they have a persistence that, with some delays, enables them to learn surprisingly much.

They play the piano, swim, ride horses, play basketball, baseball, and soccer, take ballet lessons—you name it. They do chores around the house, catch the school bus on their own, help the neighbor carry groceries, feed the family pet. And someday they will grow up, hold jobs, and be contributing members of society.

These things *will* happen. Your hard work with your baby and child will be rewarded. Just remember that your baby is first and foremost a child. With your tenacity, encouragement, and—most of all—your love, that child is going to blossom.

While your child is growing and learning, so are you. If you gain nothing else, you will at least develop a point of view that might be somewhat different from one you've held before. To some it will seem slightly askew; but it is nothing more than rejoicing at life's small victories.

For example, one particular family had worked so diligently to expand their little girl's vocabulary. One Sunday morning as various family members were sitting around reading the paper the two-year-old lost her temper and, clearly enough to please Professor Higgins shouted, "Damn it! Damn it! Damn it!" Mother, father, brother, and sister jumped up and down for joy! Only hours later did they remember that perhaps instead of jumping they should have been saying "No-no!" But on further reflection they decided it was better to hear her say a nice clear "Damn it!" than to not hear her say anything at all.

The Future

As time passes, you will begin to look at the birth of your baby very differently. Far from the grief and despair you felt at her birth, you will feel joy and pride. You will come to see the precious little baby you originally dreamed of, and Down syndrome will take on a different—and proper—perspective.

Many parents will tell you that if you are going to have a child with a disability, be glad it's Down syndrome. Compared to many other types of disabilities, Down syndrome seems almost minimal. Children with Down syndrome are physically very capable, love and appreciate their families, and enjoy life very much. Remember, children with Down syndrome are much more *like* other children than *unlike* them.

It is important to note that the dictionary definition of the verb "to retard" is "to cause to move more slowly." Mental retardation does *not* mean "unintelligent." People who still link mental retardation with "unintelligent" are often at a loss when they meet children with Down syndrome and find they do not fit their preconceived notions. Children with Down syndrome may have some limitations, but within those limitations they are bright, inquisitive, and often surprisingly erudite.

This was not always thought to be so. Perhaps no other group of people with mental retardation has been so stigmatized. It may be that because of similar physical characteristics, it has been easy to lump them together and slap a label on them. They were automatically consigned to the bottom of the barrel. More often than not, the diagnosis of Down syndrome was a passport to an institution or a back room. Sadly, these children then lived up to the dreadful images remembered from old biology textbooks or exposés of institutional life; they became victims of a self-fulfilling prophecy.

Today there is a new generation of children with Down syndrome who are leading very different lives. This is a generation of potential. Old stereotypes are being laid to rest. Your baby is of this new generation. No one should place limits on her.

Consider the youngster who while waiting to get his hair cut in an Italian barbershop, suddenly stood up and sang out at the top of his lungs, dreadfully off key, "Figaro! Figaro! Figaro!" His mother didn't know whether to stare transfixed at the ceiling, deny all kinship and claim a quiet child in a corner as her own, or express the triumph she felt that her son could equate grand opera with a happening in his own life. The misgivings she felt about any possible ethnic misunderstanding, mixed with pride in her son's perception, were dissolved when barbers and patrons alike applauded as the impromptu performer climbed into the barber chair.

There is no getting away from it. Although generalizations are as difficult with kids who have Down syndrome as with any others, the child with Down syndrome is often "the personality kid." Endearing, compassionate, exuberant, often stubborn, just as often mischievous, the child with Down syndrome has a genius for bringing out the best in people. Families who think they will never smile again find that life centers around their child in a joyous way they could not have dreamed possible when the baby was born.

Your baby has Down syndrome. It's a fact of this fresh little life and of yours. The birth of this baby has given a new challenge to your life and quite possibly a new set of values as well. A different dimension has been added, partly frightening and partly sad, but also beautiful. You wish with all your heart that your baby had been born "normal"; you wish it for her and you wish it for you. But you don't have time to dwell on that. Right now, above all else, your baby *needs* you. Someday, probably as you are giving a bath, spooning in the spinach, patting up a good burp, or even walking the floor in the wee hours, it will hit you how very much *you* need your baby.

Parent Statements

I found out Amanda had Down syndrome right after she was born. I asked the doctors what it was, because I wasn't real familiar with it, and they said there would be some mental retardation. They were encouraging; they told me she'd be able to read, and they gave me a little brief of what to expect. But I was just so happy about having a baby that it didn't really hit me right away. I'd seen her when she was born; she was really healthy and everything.

We were not told right away. There were a couple days there where we actually hoped that he didn't have Down syndrome. We knew just enough to be very worried.

My family and relatives were very supportive. Initially my husband took the news harder than I did, but he rallied really well. And then we had lots of support from close friends and our church. I was disappointed, of course. I didn't want her to have Down syndrome. For a long time, when I would think about what she might grow up to be, I'd have a really hard time with it. But it never struck me as being a terrible tragedy. See, everybody was very accepting; nobody said "Oh no, this is awful." They were very encouraging. Not one person acted negatively. It was "Well, it's too bad but, hey, it's great you had your baby, and that's wonderful."

We didn't want to tell anyone that our daughter might have Down syndrome until the karyotyping confirmed it. So, the first few days she was home, we told people she was still in the hospital with jaundice. We didn't want anyone to come over to see her; we didn't want to have to put on happy faces when we were so despondent. We almost got caught in our lie when my brother brought a casserole over for us. We hid the baby in the walk-in closet, and then held our breaths hoping she wouldn't cry and give us away. We had to be kind of rude to my brother to get him to leave. He understood later, and we can all laugh about it now, but at the time, we never thought we'd laugh about anything again.

My initial reaction was total shock, but soon after, I wanted information. What did this mean, what is going on, why? But we didn't really push the why. We wanted information, but realized that we had to hold together for Laurie, even though she was this minute-old baby. And we had to be together for other people who were going to take our lead on how we reacted and accepted her. If we acted unaccepting, so would everybody else. Or if we tried to deny it in any way—or tried to delay it. We didn't know the best way to explain it to people, because there is no best way. You just have to say it.

When the doctors told us at the hospital that our son had Down syndrome, we both just thought the world opened up and swallowed us right then.

Our whole approach from day one has been that we accepted this right away and the question was not "why was it?" or "whose fault was it?" or "why did we deserve this?" but "what do we have to do to make her the best person she can be?"

❧❧❧❧❧❧❧❧

I wanted people to say congratulations, and they didn't. It was like my baby had died.

❧❧❧❧❧❧❧❧

I kept wanting people to act like they were just happy that I had a baby. You know, not like it was terrible that he was born.

❧❧❧❧❧❧❧❧

We thought it would be harder to tell people later. So we told everyone right away. And the response from family and friends was just really wonderful. They came to see us. They showered her with everything under the sun. To us it really meant, "She's an important person and we're glad she's here." Because that's how we felt.

❧❧❧❧❧❧❧❧

Everybody was sympathetic. I don't remember any harsh or negative comments. Everybody was just as nice as they could be. They didn't treat him or us as weird. They didn't always know how to approach him, but I put myself in their position. I'd feel awkward too, so I wasn't offended.

❧❧❧❧❧❧❧❧

After my daughter's Down syndrome was confirmed, I called my sister to tell her the news. She heard me out, then said, "When you said you had bad news, I thought you were going to tell me that Hope has something really awful like a fatal disease." That kind of put things in perspective for me.

❧❧❧❧❧❧❧❧

Most of our relatives have been very positive. With a couple exceptions, most of them have more than met our expectations and really looked on our son just as a new relative. But one did not. One of Josh's cousins must have been told, "This child has Down syndrome, he's different," because the child acted very differently towards him. That hurt us a lot.

Pone of the cousins must have been told, "This child has

The first person we told about our daughter's Down syndrome reacted by saying, "Oh really?" My husband thought that was an inappropriate response. But really, what would an appropriate response be? You don't want someone to say "That's terrible!" And you don't want them to say "That's great!" I truly don't know what *I'd* say if one of my friends had a baby with Down syndrome. You can't hold people's initial responses against them.

My wife was most upset about Christopher having Down syndrome and I think particularly because we'd been so hopeful that it wouldn't be. You see, we'd been told by several doctors who were really experts, just on the basis of a quick examination, that it probably wasn't Down syndrome. It made it even worse because we had held out hope for a long time. And after we found out, the first things that came to mind were the worst images because we really didn't know—we knew more bad things about Down syndrome than good. We didn't know the mitigating factors.

I've talked with a lot of parents who weren't as lucky as we were. They didn't have a diagnosis of their child until the preschool years because it wasn't a clear-cut diagnosis like Down syndrome. They're just now beginning to realize that their child has mental retardation. It's much easier when you know from the beginning what you have to deal with. The other parents were always holding out the hope that their child would end up normal.

~~~~~~~~~

The nicest times are when people treat Chris like any other baby. They say, "Oh, what a beautiful baby!" And that makes us proud because he is a beautiful baby, and we feel very happy about that. One time we were in an airport and someone came up to us and said, "Down syndrome?" When I said yes, he said, "Wonderful children. I've got one myself." It was nice of him.

~~~~~~~~~

One part of me was extremely sad—I couldn't stop crying. It took me a year to stop crying. And the other side of me wanted to be really happy and take her for walks and enjoy my new baby. It was a strange situation. Other people had a hard time because outwardly I probably looked really together and happy. Since then, some people have said to me that it was really weird. And it was.

~~~~~~~~~

After our daughter was diagnosed with Down syndrome, several people told me that they thought I was a strong person who could handle this. I know they meant well, but they made me feel worse. I felt like they were minimizing the enormity of the problem I faced. If this was something I could deal with, as utterly helpless and devastated as I felt, then they must really think that finding out that your kid has Down syndrome is no big deal.

~~~~~~~~~

Sometimes I have feelings of resentment. I don't think against anyone specifically, but when I go to the grocery store and I see people all concerned over some little thing like the kid's diaper not being on right, I feel like saying, "Come on, give me a break, save it for something really serious."

We weren't particularly interested in why the cells didn't separate properly. We didn't really look back. Various people go from doctor to doctor and ask, "Why did this happen to me?" But we figure, he's here, he's got forty-seven chromosomes. Nothing is ever going to change that, we'll deal with it as it is.

I think it made a big impact when people wanted to extend condolences, and we came back at them very positive and optimistic. We had to let them know that this wasn't a sad moment and they kind of backed off with their condolences.

My reaction now when I see a baby with Down syndrome is, I think, "Oh, how nice." But it makes me feel strange if somebody says, "Oh they are wonderful children," because that's stereotyping. They aren't all wonderful any more than any other children are all wonderful.

One of the things that I remember right after she was born, and it kind of irked me, was that lots of people acted as if it was a real tragedy, like it was a real sorrowful moment in our lives and they had to apologize for us. The flowers came in like it was a wake, not a birth. But I remember one guy who came in and he was all grins and congratulations, and he shook my hand. It dawned on me that this guy's reaction was different. He was reacting the way someone's supposed to react when you give birth to a child. That put everybody else's reactions into perspective.

I think it takes a long time for parents to accept other people looking at their child. And now that I've had another child, I realize that people look at *any* baby. They don't just look at the baby because she has Down syndrome or has a disability. People stare at babies.

I still have trouble telling people about my son. You know, I say I have a child and I think to myself, now do I have to tell them he has Down syndrome? I don't want to introduce that to people I don't know. I don't want to say he has mental retardation, he's got Down syndrome. That's something I still have to work through my system.

My daughter is going on two, and I still think about the fact that she has Down syndrome every day. I'll think, "Oh, she really looks (or doesn't look) like she has Down syndrome right now." Or, "I wonder if she's doing that because she has Down syndrome?" Or, "Wow—she seems so smart and inquisitive; how could she have Down syndrome?" I don't feel especially sad when I think these things, but I guess I haven't really accepted her Down syndrome, either.

One day I took Laurie to the park. There was a couple there with a little boy around two and his grandmother. The little boy kept pointing at us. He'd run over to Laurie from a distance and pull her hair and run away. Our little girl just started screaming—naturally. The grandmother looked back and said, "Well, that little girl is retarded." I just thought, "Well, your little boy isn't very nice." Of course she was screaming—her hair was being pulled. It took me by surprise, but I just thought, "Why should I say anything? It won't change anything." It was the first time that's ever happened to me.

I had a particularly hard time with one neighbor. She had a little girl just about the same age as mine. I really had a hard time when that girl first sat up, when she crawled, when she walked. She was talking a blue streak in a year, and that was really hard for me. It took me a long time to like that little girl—isn't that awful?

~ ~ ~ ~ ~ ~ ~ ~ ~

One time a woman came up to us and said, "Oh, what a nice little child. Just think, he'll always be childlike. What a wonderful thing, he'll never grow up." I thought it was funny because she was trying very hard to say something nice and yet she completely misunderstood.

~ ~ ~ ~ ~ ~ ~ ~ ~

When he was smaller, not many people said anything to me about the baby. We were at an evening dinner, and the baby was with us, and a woman invited us to her new babies parent group that she'd just started. When I said he had Down syndrome, she looked like she had a hot potato. She looked sort of horrified as if she were recoiling, and then she never got in touch with us afterwards. I always felt a bit bitter, and I thought she was a bit stupid anyway, to have that kind of reaction.

~ ~ ~ ~ ~ ~ ~ ~ ~

I've run into strange reactions on the part of parents whose kids aren't quite perfect in some minor way. I have a little bit of impatience, but then I think they're just families who haven't experienced the full range of perspective. People get all upset because their kid has an ear infection. When your kid has open-heart surgery and some other kid has a minor infection, you think well, no big deal.

~ ~ ~ ~ ~ ~ ~ ~ ~

Now that Chris is older, people ask, "How old is that lovely baby?" and I say twenty months, and they say "Ten?" And I say twenty, and they say "Oh." And then they say "Can he say his name?" because he is so old and he doesn't walk yet and he doesn't talk well, so people notice. I don't feel embarrassed, just a bit withdrawn.

Some people acted like the baby was dead. I didn't get a lot of presents for him—not that you care about the presents themselves, but I cared about what it meant. My aunt didn't even tell her friends we had a baby.

Maybe you think you and your baby would be better off if he died. Believe me, you wouldn't. In addition to having a baby with Down syndrome, I had a baby (without Down syndrome) who died. Dying is indescribably worse than Down syndrome. When you have a child with Down syndrome, there is always hope: hope that he will learn new skills; hope that new and better treatments will be developed; hope that society will become more accepting of people with disabilities. When you have a child who dies, all hope dies with him. Nothing ever changes for the better; all you're left with is sad, fading memories of a little person who could have grown up to do great things, but was robbed of the chance.

Initially we thought there would be a million decisions to make right away, but we found that the decisions were spread over a long period of time, like with any other child. The decisions aren't knocking at your door every day.

Three

Medical Concerns and Treatments

Chahira Kozma, M.D.*

Although babies with Down syndrome can be just as healthy as any other children, they can also have special medical problems. Even though some of these problems can be quite serious, the good news is that medical treatments have improved substantially, and the vast majority of babies with Down syndrome grow up healthy and active.

As with other characteristics of children with Down syndrome, exactly how the extra number 21 chromosome causes medical problems is not known. But, as discussed below, new discoveries in the field of molecular genetics are shedding some light on the complex relation between genes and human development and diseases.

In the past, the medical problems associated with Down syndrome resulted in shortened life spans and premature deaths. Sometimes decisions were made not to perform life-saving surgery. Today, however, there are advanced medical treatments for virtually every medical problem babies with Down syndrome may have.

In the early 1930s, the estimated life expectancy of people with Down syndrome was only nine years. Many died very

---

*   Dr. Chahira Kozma is Assistant Professor of Pediatrics and a Clinical Geneticist at Georgetown University Medical Center in Washington, D.C.

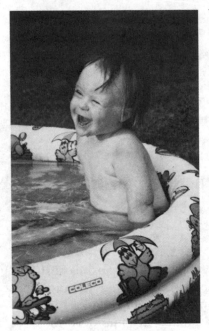

young from heart problems that could not be cured at that time. By 1990, however, improved medical care had increased the average life span to more than 30 years, and now an increasing number survive to over 50 years of age. Just as important, the quality of life for people with Down syndrome has improved dramatically.

All babies have a chance of developing any number of diseases or conditions, but parents of newborns are usually not presented with the statistics as soon as their baby is born. Yet those statistics exist for every infant. Every baby has a possibility of developing heart problems, vision problems, hearing problems, infections, or anything else you care to name. But when your baby has Down syndrome, doctors come to tell you the statistics. It may seem insensitive and unfair, but the reason for raising the issue so early is simply that babies with Down syndrome have a higher incidence of certain medical problems and these problems are usually best dealt with as soon as possible.

Along with the dramatic increase in knowledge about Down syndrome and the medical conditions often associated with it, new methods for well-child health care have developed. Today, specialized clinics as well as your pediatrician can set up a well-child care program that includes screening, early identification, treatment, and prevention of the medical conditions and complications associated with Down syndrome. This kind of program can go a long way toward ensuring your baby stays as healthy as possible.

This chapter reviews the medical problems babies with Down syndrome may have, and the treatment of those problems. Because early detection and treatment is often crucial, learning the basic facts about medical conditions can help you spot problems, ask the right questions, communicate well with doctors, and make important decisions.

As you read, remember that not every baby has the medical problems covered in this chapter. Some have none, some have a few, and some have many. These are conditions that babies with Down syndrome statistically have higher chances of developing than do other babies, and these conditions could hamper early development. And remember also that in medicine, forewarned is often forearmed.

Heart Defects

About 40 to 45 percent of babies with Down syndrome are born with heart defects. Heart defects that exist at birth are often called *congenital heart defects* ("congenital" means present at birth). Prior to the development of advanced cardiac surgery, many of these defects led to death. Recent surgical advances make it possible to repair most defects, even those once thought to be hopeless. These dramatic advances have resulted in improved survival and quality of life for babies with Down syndrome who have heart defects.

Before discussing the common heart defects babies with Down syndrome may have, let's review some general information about the heart. The heart is a strong pump made of muscle. It is about the size of your fist. The heart has four chambers which are separated by walls made of heart muscle. Valves between the chambers open and close to allow blood to flow in only the correct direction. Blood is pumped into and out of the heart via the major vessels (arteries and veins) that are attached to it. The two upper chambers are called the *atria*, and the two lower chambers are called the *ventricles*. Blood that has been circulating in the body and is low in oxygen returns to the right side of the heart, where it is pumped to the lungs. In the lungs, the blood receives fresh oxygen and returns to the left side of the heart, where it is pumped into general circulation, delivering oxygen to all parts of the body.

When a baby has a heart defect, there may be a hole in the walls between the chambers. The result is that too much blood is pumped to the lungs and not enough blood is pumped to the rest of the body. Consequently, the body does not get enough oxygen-carrying blood. In addition, because a hole can disrupt the flow of blood within the heart and allow blood to pool, this condition can raise the risk of serious cardiac infections.

There are several types of heart defects. The most common in babies with Down syndrome is called an *atrioventricular canal defect* or *AV canal*, as it is commonly called. It is also sometimes referred to as an *endocardial cushion defect*. An AV canal is a large hole in the center of the heart. This means that the walls between the two upper chambers (the atria) and the two lower chambers (the ventricles), as well as the valves between them, may be deformed. This large opening in the center of the heart allows the red oxygenated blood to mix with low-oxygen blood and return to the lungs. This forces the heart to pump an extra amount of blood to the lungs. This extra effort in turn causes the heart to enlarge. In addition, the body receives less oxygen since it receives red blood that is mixed with low-oxygen blood.

Most infants with an AV canal grow very slowly and remain small. Because of the high volume of blood that is pumped to the lungs, high blood pressure may occur there, resulting in damage to the lungs and blood vessels. Surgical repair of an AV canal usually restores blood circulation to normal.

Another common heart defect in babies with Down syndrome is the *ventricular septal defect (VSD)*. A VSD is a large opening between the ventricles in which, as with AV canals, oxygenated and deoxygenated blood mix, resulting in similar problems to AV canals, including low blood oxygen levels, an enlarged heart, and high blood pressure. There are other less common heart defects including holes between the two upper chambers (*atrial septal defect* or *ASD*), problems with the heart valves, and defects in the major arteries attached to the heart.

Heart defects are serious problems. In their most severe form, they can threaten your baby's life soon after birth and require emergency corrective surgery. Even defects that do not need immediate surgery can drastically shorten life if left untreated. If, because of an untreated heart defect, excess blood is continually pumped to the lungs, high pressure in the blood vessels in the lungs (called *pulmonary hypertension*) will result. Over time, the blood vessels will become scarred, and, if not treated soon enough, will eventually become so narrow that not enough blood can reach the lungs. This condition is fatal.

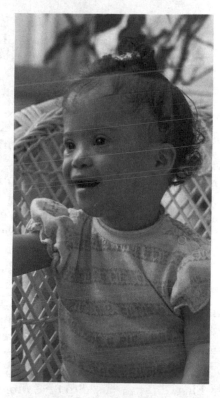

Whenever a baby with Down syndrome is born, he needs to be examined carefully by a pediatrician and a clinical geneticist for any signs or symptoms of heart defects. Most heart defects are detected at birth, but occasionally, the defect may not be detected until a few weeks or months of age. One common diagnostic technique is the *echocardiogram*, a painless test that uses high-frequency sound waves to create an image of the heart. It should be a part of the routine evaluation of any baby with Down syndrome.

If your baby is found to have a heart defect (or even if it is suspected), he needs to be evaluated further by a *pediatric cardiologist*, a doctor who specializes in heart defects in children. The pediatric cardiologist should examine your baby immediately after birth and continue to monitor him closely for some time afterwards. The pediatric cardiologist can assess your baby by physical examination, heart x-rays, *electrocardiogram* (ECG), and echocardiogram. ECG records the electrical activity of the heart. These tests help your doctor assess the structure and function of the heart. One technique, called *cardiac catheterization*, allows doctors to view the inside of the heart to evaluate in detail any defect. Since this test is invasive (it is a surgical procedure), it is not done routinely. It is typically done when a baby is in heart failure (discussed below) or immediately before cardiac surgery.

After carefully examining your baby, the pediatric cardiologist will advise you on appropriate treatments. If surgery is recommended, a pediatric heart surgeon and your cardiologist will discus their recommendations with you and answer your questions. Repeated examinations are crucial for continuous monitoring and control of any cardiac problems your baby may have.

Babies with heart defects may show symptoms of what is called "heart failure." Heart failure does *not* mean the heart is stopping, but rather that it cannot keep up with the body's needs. The clearest symptoms are poor feeding, a change in color during feeding, poor growth, and labored breathing. Sometimes the baby's skin may turn blue (*cyanosis*), especially during times of feeding or physical exertion. Other signs include accelerated breathing and frequent upper respiratory infections. Children with heart failure need to be very closely monitored by their doctors, parents, and teachers.

There are two ways heart defects are treated by doctors. First, drugs are used to treat minor defects and to help babies with more serious defects survive until they are ready for surgery. For example, drugs that reduce the amount of water in the body are used to ease the heart's job. These drugs, called *diuretics*, help the body expel extra fluid in order to reduce the amount of blood the heart must pump. Digoxin is also a commonly used drug that helps the heart to contract with more force and function more efficiently.

Second, open heart surgery may be necessary to correct a defect. The decision to operate to fix a heart defect depends on multiple factors, including complexity of the defect, any related problems, your child's age and weight, and psychological and social considerations. For instance, a baby with a severe AV canal may be operated on early in the first year of life, whereas a small VSD with minimal symptoms may be closed at a few years of age. Studies show that currently there is approximately a 75 percent survival rate following surgical repair of an AV canal, and a greater survival rate in those with a VSD or a hole between just the upper chambers of the heart. Following successful surgery, an improvement in heart function, growth, and development can be expected. Most children who have heart defects repaired successfully go on to lead healthy lives.

According to the American Heart Association, if your baby has a heart defect, he can be best served at a center specializing in caring for children with these conditions. Specialists in these centers include pediatric cardiologists, cardiothoracic surgeons, intensive-care experts, and a skilled support team. Heart centers and hospitals specializing in pediatric surgery exist across the country. It is important, however, to find the right specialist for your child's particular surgery. As a parent, do not hesitate to inquire about the experience of the heart surgery team and the success of their operations. Look for a cardiac surgeon with experience in pediatrics for whom this type of surgery is routine. The Resource Guide at the end of the book contains listings of Down syndrome clinics, university hospitals, and organizations that can refer you to the right doctor.

For over one hundred years doctors have known that heart defects are associated with Down syndrome. In the past, there was little, if anything, that could be done in the way of treatment. Fortunately, children with Down syndrome and heart defects can be successfully treated early in life, resulting in increased longevity and improved quality of life. Today, the prognosis for most babies is greatly improved.

Gastrointestinal Problems

Babies with Down syndrome have a 10 to 12 percent chance of being born with some type of congenital malformation of the gastrointestinal (digestive) system. The most commonly encountered anomaly is a narrowing or blockage of the small intestine, called *duodenal atresia*. In fact, whenever duodenal atresia is diagnosed prenatally or in the newborn period, there is a 20 to 40 percent chance that the fetus or the newborn has Down syndrome. Other common gastrointestinal anomalies include: 1) *imperforate anus*, the absence of an anal opening; 2) *pyloric stenosis*,

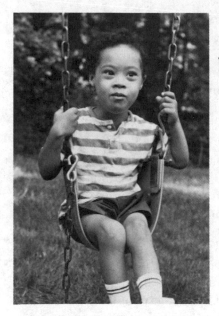

obstruction of the outlet of the stomach; 3) *tracheo-esophageal fistula*, an abnormal opening between the trachea (wind pipe) and the esophagus (food pipe); and 4) *Hirschsprung's disease*, the absence of nerves in the colon (large intestine). Some of these conditions, such as tracheo-esophageal fistula, are serious and require immediate surgical correction.

Gastrointestinal problems usually appear right after birth. The symptoms often include poor feeding, vomiting, swollen abdomen, lack of stools, or pneumonia. The malformations can be successfully corrected surgically, but need to be recognized promptly. Following surgery, your baby will be able to digest formula and other foods normally.

If your baby has a congenital defect of the intestinal tract, your pediatrician should consult with a pediatric surgeon and refer you to a pediatric center where this type of surgery is performed routinely.

Respiratory Problems

In the past, one of the most common causes of early death in children with Down syndrome was respiratory infection. Today, however, with modern antibiotics and better general medical care, the majority of respiratory infections can be treated well. Respiratory problems sometimes occur more frequently in children with Down syndrome for several reasons. These include poor coughing ability, poor handling of oral secretions, and abnormal immune systems. Other factors include low muscle tone and regurgitation of food from the stomach into the esophagus and throat (commonly called *gastroesophageal reflux*). A respiratory infection is usually a viral or bacterial infection of the nasal passages, throat, bronchial tubes, or lungs. *Bronchitis* (an infection of the bronchial tubes) and *pneumonia* (an infection of the lungs) are both serious respiratory infections requiring medical attention. Respiratory infections are more often seen in children who have congenital heart defects and complications like congestive heart failure and excess fluid in the lungs.

Another type of respiratory problem that is more common in babies and children with Down syndrome is *sleep apnea,* or temporary stopping of breathing. Sleep apnea occurs more often among premature babies, babies with certain medical problems, and babies with Down syndrome. Among babies with Down syndrome, sleep apnea is usually due to upper airway obstruction. The upper airways can be obstructed by large adenoids, large tonsils, large tongue, or a combination of the above. Symptoms include noisy breathing, frequent apnea, fitful sleep, and snoring. Children with these symptoms have difficulty in draining fluids from the middle ear to the throat, and, more importantly, have decreased oxygen levels in the brain, lungs, and the rest of the body during sleep. If you suspect your child has upper airway obstruction, notify your pediatrician or consult an ear, nose, and throat specialist. Children who have upper airway obstruction can often be treated successfully by removing the adenoids, tonsils, or both.

Vision

Children's eyes are not fully developed at birth. In fact, all babies are nearsighted during their first few weeks of life. Their sight and eye control will usually improve, but at first they do not see very well. For this reason it is often difficult to determine if there is a problem with a child's sight. Most children with Down syndrome have the same quality of sight as other children and develop the same control of their eyes, but because eyesight can affect other facets of development, it is especially important to make sure your child's eyesight is normal as early as possible.

Close to 70 percent of children with Down syndrome have some type of eye problems. Early eye examinations are crucial

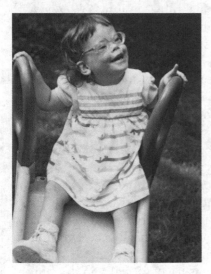

to detect and treat eye problems because the majority of eye problems are correctable. Early examination will ensure that poor eyesight is spotted and treated and does not interfere with your child's development or cause additional problems. A pediatric ophthalmologist—a physician specializing in the eyes and eye diseases of children—should be consulted in the first year of your baby's life. Earlier evaluation may be necessary if you or your pediatrician suspect a problem. Periodic eye evaluation every one or two years is recommended thereafter.

Vision problems that children with Down syndrome may have are similar to those other children have. However, they occur at a higher rate in children with Down syndrome. The problems include crossed eyes, nearsightedness, farsightedness, astigmatism, cataracts, and tear duct obstruction. Each of these problems can be detected and corrected early so as not to hinder development. Let's briefly review the types of visual problems and their treatment:

Crossed Eyes. Crossed eyes, also known as strabismus, occurs in approximately 57 percent of babies and children with Down syndrome. The condition results from an imbalance in the eye muscles; the muscles pull the eyes in different directions. As a result, the eyes tend to turn (or *deviate*) in or out.

If an eye is crossed or deviated, it will result in blurred vision. To prevent the blurred vision, the brain may ignore the signals sent from the deviated eye. If signals from the eye are ignored long enough, the eye will fail to develop good vision and can even become completely blind. This condition is called *am-*

blyopia or lazy eye. To prevent amblyopia, it is important to evaluate strabismus early and prescribe treatment which may include corrective glasses, patching of the healthy eye, surgery, or a combination of them. With early detection and treatment, most deviated eyes can be straightened and amblyopia prevented.

Nearsightedness and Farsightedness. Nearsightedness and farsightedness are common problems in children with Down syndrome. These conditions occur at a rate of 20 to 22 percent among people with Down syndrome.

Eyes are like cameras; they take in a picture through the lens and display it on the retina. This process is called *refraction.* The shape of your child's eye determines whether his refraction is focused or blurred. If your child has a refractory problem, it means that images are not projected onto the retina clearly. With nearsightedness, also called *myopia,* there is poor vision for distant objects, and children tend to hold books, toys, or other objects very close to their eyes. In farsightedness, also called *hypermetropia,* there is poor vision for close objects. Children with these conditions often lack interest in books and games and have headaches or crossed eyes. These conditions can be treated quite well with glasses or contact lenses.

Astigmatism. *Astigmatism* is another problem with refraction that is common among people with Down syndrome; it occurs in about 22 percent of people with Down syndrome. In astigmatism, there is a slight irregularity in the shape of the eyeball. This irregularity prevents light rays from focusing on a single point on the retina as they do in normally-shaped eyes. The result is that blurred images are formed. Symptoms of astigmatism include headache, eye pain, and fatigue. Like other refraction errors, astigmatism can be treated with corrective lenses.

Cataracts. In children and adults with Down syndrome, sometimes the lens of one or both eyes becomes cloudy. The result is deteriorating vision. The treatment today is surgery to replace the damaged lens with a new one. Rare in young children, this condition is slightly more common in children with Down syndrome.

Blocked tear ducts. Obstruction of the tear duct (called *naso lacrimal duct obstruction*), is found in about 15 percent of babies with Down syndrome (and is quite common in other children as well). It results in excess tearing or infection of the tear duct. Massaging the tear duct, in combination with eye drops for treatment of any infection, is usually successful in opening the duct. Occasionally minor surgery is necessary to clear up the condition.

Hearing

Infants hear and listen from the moment of birth. As parents quickly learn, they respond to loud sounds by startling, jumping, or crying. Soon babies learn to recognize and respond to your voice and tell the difference between the voices of their siblings and the voices of others.

The development of speech and language depends on hearing. Because untreated hearing loss can lead to delayed speech, delayed language development, and social and emotional problems, it is very important to detect and treat hearing loss as early as possible. If your child has a mild hearing loss, he may have trouble hearing certain sounds, or hearing in certain situations. If he has a moderate to severe hearing loss, he may have trouble in many situations. If he has a profound loss, he will be able to hear little or nothing around him. Numerous studies report that between 40 and 60 percent of babies and children with Down syndrome have a hearing loss. The hearing loss is usually great enough to affect language acquisition and educational achievement.

There are several types of hearing loss. A *conductive hearing loss* occurs when sound is not able to travel efficiently through the ear canal, ear drum, or the tiny bones of the middle ear. Conductive hearing loss can be caused by frequent colds, allergies, or buildup of fluid in the middle ear. A *sensorineural hearing loss* occurs when there is damage to the inner ear or to the nerves leading from the inner ear to the brain. There is also a mixed type of hearing loss, when a combination of conductive and sensorineural hearing losses are present.

One of the most common and challenging causes of hearing loss in children with Down syndrome is middle ear fluid. Children with Down syndrome may have this problem sooner and more often than others because of frequent colds, smaller ear passages, low muscle tone, and allergies. The middle ear is connected to the back of the throat by a small tube called the *eustachian tube*. This tube is supposed to drain fluid from the ear into the back of the throat. It can become blocked, resulting in increased risk of infection and in retention of fluid in the middle ear. Fluid in the middle ear interferes with the vibration of the eardrum, which reduces hearing sensitivity. The hearing loss should be temporary, but may come and go repeatedly; when the fluid clears, freeing the eardrum, hearing should improve. If the fluid remains in the middle ear for a long time, however, significant hearing loss can occur. This hearing loss can occur whether or not infection is present. That is, your child may show no signs of discomfort and still have enough fluid to cause a hearing loss. For these children, sounds may be muffled and language development may be delayed.

An audiologist, a professional who specializes in assessing hearing, can evaluate your child's hearing accurately at any age. In fact, even newborn babies can have accurate hearing tests. *Auditory brainstem response* (ABR), a test that measures electronically the brain's reception of sounds, is recommended prior to your baby's discharge from the hospital nursery. ABR can be given until six months of age. For infants older than six months, tests that require a response from your child can be used. Another common test that is used to evaluate middle ear function is known as *tympanometry*. This procedure is used to test the function of the eardrum and to detect fluid in the middle ear.

Your child should receive a hearing evaluation each year until 3 years of age and every other year thereafter. Most children with Down syndrome have very small ear canals, making it difficult to examine them properly with the instruments found in the pediatric office. Consequently, it may be necessary for your child to see an Ear, Nose, and Throat (ENT) physician to examine his eardrums using a microscopic otoscope. If your child has abnormal hearing tests or accumulation of fluid in the middle ear, he should see an ENT physician.

Doctors typically use antibiotics or decongestants or a combination of both to treat ear infections and fluid in the middle ear. If your child has recurrent infections and persistent fluid in his middle ear, his doctor may implant small tubes through the eardrum that help drain the fluid and return normal function to the middle ear. Implanting the tubes is a relatively minor outpatient surgery.

Children with Down syndrome who have hearing losses that cannot be corrected medically should be referred to an experienced audiologist for follow up. Depending on the degree of hearing loss, the audiologist will determine the most appropriate way to handle the problem. If your child has a mild hearing loss, suggestions can be given for communication at home as well as school. If a moderate or severe hearing loss is detected, the audiologist may recommend amplification devices, such as hearing aids. Hearing aids are usually effective in restoring normal hearing or near-normal hearing. Your audiologist can make sure the hearing aids fit correctly and are comfortable. He or she will also teach you how to take care of the device, and can design a program for helping your child get used to wearing them.

Hearing is vital for your child's development. Children cannot learn to speak well if they cannot hear well. Even a mild hearing loss can affect speech development. So, make sure your baby can hear normally. With early detection, medical care, and, if necessary, hearing aids, there is every reason to expect your child with Down syndrome to hear normally.

Thyroid Problems

The thyroid is a tiny gland located in the neck. The hormones it produces play very important roles in regulating how the body processes and uses sugar, fat, and vitamins.

Doctors have found that babies with Down syndrome are more likely to have a thyroid problem, especially low thyroid production, called *hypothyroidism*. Depending on the study cited, 13 to 54 percent of children and adults with Down syndrome have hypothyroidism. Hypothyroidism occurs when the thyroid gland decreases or stops secreting thyroid hormone. The symptoms of hypothyroidism include decreased energy level, slowed physical and mental development in young children, thickening of the skin, constipation, and sleepiness.

Hypothyroidism is a potentially serious problem and, if undetected or untreated, can cause developmental delays and other serious complications. Today, however, hypothyroidism can be controlled with medicine. Babies with Down syndrome should be screened for thyroid problems every year because symptoms of the disease are often not apparent until the damage is done. Only blood tests will reveal if there is a problem *before* the symptoms of hypothyroidism appear. These tests can be performed by your baby's pediatrician.

Orthopedic Problems

The overall low muscle tone and increased looseness of the ligaments between the bones make children and adults with Down syndrome prone to a number of orthopedic problems. These problems are often encountered after infancy.

Atlantoaxial Instability. Perhaps the most serious complication resulting from low muscle tone and joint laxity is the instability of the two upper bones of the back. This condition, known as *atlantoaxial instability,* occurs in about 10 percent of children and adults with Down syndrome. The lax joints allow for excessive movement between the two upper vertebrae, especially when the neck is extended or bent. Children who have this condition run a risk of spinal cord injury because their two upper vertebrae allow too much bending of the spinal cord.

In a small percentage of children with atlantoaxial instability, about 1 or 2 percent, the upper vertebrae slips, compressing and damaging the spinal cord. The symptoms of spinal cord compression from atlantoaxial instability are fatigue during walking, difficulties in walking, progressive clumsiness, neck pain, head tilt, and contraction of the muscles of the neck. The majority of children with atlantoaxial instability, however, have no symptoms at all. That is why detection of the condition is im-

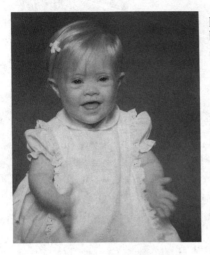

portant. This is done routinely by x-rays of the neck between the ages of 4 and 5 years.

Children with atlantoaxial instability need to avoid contact sports, somersaults, trampoline exercises, and other activities that may lead to excess stress of the neck. If your child has atlantoaxial instability, he needs to be under the supervision of an orthopedist and to be monitored carefully by his primary care doctor. The small number of children with Down syndrome who develop symptoms of spinal cord damage need surgery to fuse unstable vertebras. This surgery does not significantly affect movement or development.

Children with Down syndrome like to be active, as do all children. Many participate in vigorous activity and sports programs. To guide you in supervising your child's activity, the American Academy of Pediatrics recommends: 1) all children with Down syndrome who wish to participate in sports involving possible trauma to the head and neck should have an x-ray to assess the cervical region; 2) children with Down syndrome should have an x-ray of the spine routinely between the ages of four and five; 3) children with any signs of instability should be restricted from strenuous activity and surgical stabilization should be considered; and 4) children with Down syndrome who have no evidence of instability may participate in all sports.

Other Orthopedic Problems. The most common orthopedic problems children with Down syndrome have are abnormal toeing in of the foot (called *metatarsus varus*) and flat feet (called *pes planus*). These deformities can cause pain and difficulty in walking. These problems result from the loose joints children with Down syndrome have. They are typically treated with corrective shoes, orthopedic inserts and, if necessary, surgery. Another common orthopedic problem is instability of the kneecap (called *patellar instability*). The symptoms of kneecap instability include pain, swelling, and inability to walk when the kneecap pops out of joint. This problem can be corrected with surgery.

Dental Concerns

Children with Down syndrome have a variety of dental problems, including missing teeth, delayed tooth eruption, and misshapen teeth. These problems generally do not delay development or cause serious medical problems. On the other hand, periodontal diseases (gum diseases), which are very common in children with Down syndrome, can lead to loss of teeth. Aggressive dental hygiene is very important to reduce or prevent periodontal diseases. This includes daily brushing and flossing, reduced intake of refined sugars, good dietary habits, regular visits to the dentist, fluoride applications, and treatment of cavities. It helps a great deal to find a pediatric dentist in your community with experience and interest in working with children with Down syndrome.

Leukemia

Leukemia is a type of cancer that attacks white blood cells. White blood cells fight infection, and are critical for health. The incidence of leukemia among people with Down syndrome is about one percent. That is 15 to 20 times higher than in the general population.

Although leukemia is a very serious disease, treatment using chemotherapy, radiation therapy, and bone marrow transplants, has improved dramatically, and many patients can now be cured. More and more children survive leukemia, especially when the disease is detected early. If your baby or child is healthy, he does not need to be evaluated for leukemia on a regular basis. It is only if you or your doctor become concerned about certain symptoms such as pallor, easy bruising, unexplained fever, fatigue, or other symptoms that your child will need to be checked with the appropriate blood test.

Weight

At birth, babies with Down syndrome usually are of average weight. Initially, your baby may feed and gain weight slowly because low muscle tone makes eating more exhausting or because of a medical problem such as a heart defect. After infancy, weight gain usually is normal, but obesity can become a problem. Researchers have found that approximately 30 percent of children with Down syndrome develop obesity.

In the past, many children with Down syndrome were overweight. This was due to a number of causes. Children with Down syndrome were less active and given fewer opportunities for active play. Also, other problems—such as low muscle tone, low thyroid function, and heart defects—hindered activity. Thus, the familiar equation of too many calories and not enough activity equalled obesity.

Today there is no reason why children with Down syndrome who are in good health cannot maintain normal weight. A good diet and plenty of activity are essential, and both should be watched carefully. Consulting a nutritionist who has experience working with children with Down syndrome can be very helpful in planning menus and for recommendations with techniques to prevent overeating. The same common sense we all should follow to control our weight applies equally to children with Down syndrome.

Seizures

Scientists estimate that between 6 and 8 percent of children with Down syndrome have seizures. Seizures occur when the electrical activity of the brain is disrupted. Seizures can have many forms, ranging from convulsions to momentary lapses of attention, abnormal blinking of the eye, or unusual movements. Typically, seizures last for a brief time and then stop. They tend to be infrequent. Between seizure activities, most people are healthy.

Most types of seizures can be treated and prevented well with medications. If untreated, seizures can cause significant disabilities and interfere with development in young children. Usually, anticonvulsant medications eliminate or reduce the number of seizures. If you suspect your child is having seizures, discuss your concern with your pediatrician, who may assess your child or refer you to a neurologist.

Immunizations

Your baby needs to receive the same immunizations at the same ages as is recommended by the American Academy of Pediatrics for all children. Studies have shown no increase in complications related to vaccination among babies with Down syndrome compared to other children.

Medical Problems and Your Baby's Development

Proper medical care is essential for any baby, but particularly for yours. Medical problems left undetected or untreated can seriously slow development and prevent your child from reaching his full potential. For example, a child with poor eyesight will not be able to walk, play, or explore as he should. A child with poor hearing will not learn to talk as soon because he simply cannot hear sounds well enough. Even respiratory infections that occur too frequently can hinder development by keeping your baby inactive and away from his developmental program. For these reasons, rigorous medical care is necessary. No child deserves less.

Effective treatments are usually available for each of the medical problems children with Down syndrome may face. There are also clinics that specialize in treating children with Down syndrome. In these clinics, doctors who specialize in Down syndrome can oversee and coordinate all of the various medical services your baby may need. The many children's hospitals and university hospitals located around the country are good places to start.

Life-Saving-Surgery

Like many parents, parents of babies with Down syndrome sometimes are faced with the decision of whether to authorize life-saving surgery. A very few choose not to allow surgery, while the vast majority choose to save their baby's life.

This book and this chapter are obviously biased in favor of doing everything that can be done for babies with Down syndrome. Down syndrome alone should never be a reason for allowing a child to die. With advanced medical care and the great progress being made in education, there is no justification whatsoever to withhold necessary medical care. When you read the statements by parents at the end of this chapter you will see how natural and automatic their decisions were.

If you are facing the possibility of life-saving surgery on your baby with Down syndrome, the best advice is to first learn as much about Down syndrome as you can. Learn what that means to you and your family, but most important, learn what it means to your baby.

Concerns for the Future

Although this book focuses on the early years of life, parents often want to know what medical problems may occur later. In the past when life spans for people with Down syndrome were shorter, there simply wasn't very much information about their later life. Now, thankfully, information is building as people with Down syndrome live longer.

One issue often debated is whether people with Down syndrome lose some of their mental ability as they age. Some doctors believe that Alzheimer's disease occurs in people with Down syndrome more often than it does in other people. This is an area of intense research because it is felt that there may be a link between the extra chromosome in Down syndrome and Alzheimer's disease. Although people with Down syndrome can get the symptoms of Alzheimer's disease (gradual loss of memory and cognitive abilities, inability to manage daily life, and personality changes), research has not yet proven that the physical changes seen in people diagnosed with Alzheimer's disease always occur in people with Down syndrome.

There is very active research being conducted in this area. New medications were recently approved by the Food and Drug Administration to treat people who have Alzheimer's disease. Studies are underway to determine the effectiveness of these medications, and scientists are working hard to solve this mystery.

Children and adults with Down syndrome will benefit from medical progress in the areas of concern for the future. Remember that the problems affecting people with Down syndrome also affect others; they may just be more common in people with Down syndrome, often only slightly more common. So, as medical research discovers new cures and treatments, many problems will become less serious.

Genetics and Your Baby's Health

Parents and scientists have wondered for decades just how the extra genetic material present in Down syndrome causes the medical problems children with Down syndrome can have. Here is what is currently known: It is not that children with Down syndrome have "defective" genes; they have the same genetic material everyone else has, but they just have more of it. With new molecular testing tools, scientists are investigating how the extra genetic material in Down syndrome can cause a wide variety of medical and developmental problems, including heart defects, intestinal abnormalities, poor vision, and mental retardation. Scientists are trying to identify the genes that occupy the part of chromosome 21 that is specifically responsible for Down syndrome, and learn why three copies of these genes leads to Down syndrome.

Some of the newly discovered genes on chromosome 21 include a gene called the *amyloid Beta protein gene*. This gene controls the production of certain proteins that are present in the brains of people with early senility or Alzheimer's disease. It is possible that the extra chromosome causes overproduction of these proteins which leads to the development of Alzheimer's disease. How these genes work and their effect on the brain is an area of intensive research.

Scientists suspect other connections between the extra chromosome 21 and medical conditions. The increased incidence of cataracts and lens defects in people with Down syndrome may be explained by abnormal levels of proteins present in the lens of the eye. The gene that controls this protein is called *alpha-A-crystallin* and is located on chromosome 21. Another example of genes that are located on chromosome 21 is the *ETs-2 gene*. This gene is called an *oncogene;* it is involved in cancer or leukemia, and is important in the control of cell growth. This gene may explain why children with Down syndrome are more prone to leukemia than other children.

There are many other genes that have been located or mapped on chromosome 21 and their functions are being studied. These include the *Gart, PFKP, CBS,* and *superoxide dismutase genes* (SOD-1) which have important biochemical functions. Scientists now think that the overproduction of these genes leads to biochemical changes and damage to the body cells. Figure 10 in Chapter 1 shows some of the genes that have been mapped on chromosome 21.

The advances toward understanding the genetics of Down syndrome is growing very rapidly with exciting discoveries being made very frequently. This technology is still in its early stages, however, and it may take years to fully develop specific techniques or treatments to ameliorate or modify the effects caused by Trisomy 21. For the present and immediate future, children and adults with Down syndrome will benefit from improvements in preventive medical care, screening for medical complications, and prompt and effective treatment.

Dealing with the Medical Profession

Parents with babies who have medical problems must face additional hardships. On top of dealing with the medical problem itself, parents also have to learn to deal with the medical profession. With conflicting schedules, multiple appointments, and an entirely new language to learn, confronting a medical problem for the first time can be quite stressful. Here are a few hints:

Get the Facts. It is tremendously helpful to be able to understand what a doctor is saying to you about your child. Be it heart defects, vision problems, or just dry skin, there is a new language to learn. Learn that language by reading books, asking doctors, nurses, teachers, and other parents, and getting deeply involved in your child's care. The basic facts about a particular problem can enable you to observe your child effectively, ask the right questions, and communicate well with your child's doctor. Remember, *you* are the most critical member of the team treating your baby.

Ask Questions. When discussing your child's medical problem and treatment with a doctor, *do not* be afraid to ask questions—lots of questions. Ask until you are satisfied that you understand enough to make informed choices about your baby's medical care. Do not be intimidated. Every doctor should be able to explain medical problems and treatments in plain English. Demand full and complete explanations, including explanations of potential side effects and contingency plans. If you do not fully understand an explanation, ask to have it explained again.

Avoid Excessive Waiting. Few things are harder on parents and children than sitting in doctors' waiting rooms. It must seem that every doctor in the world runs behind schedule and that waiting around is taken for granted. Many things delay doctors, including emergencies, difficult cases, and a routinely busy schedule. Call ahead to find out if your appointment will be late. If you do have to wait, be sure to bring along something for your baby to play with. Ask for separate waiting rooms for sick and well children.

Batch Your Doctor Visits. Sometimes babies need a series of tests, such as blood tests, X-rays, and a physical examination. Try to take care of all of these things at the same time and at the same place. Try to set aside a morning or an afternoon to take your child from test to test, rather than spreading it out over days. This eliminates constant shuttling to and from your treatment center.

Watch Out for Outdated Opinions. Doctors have come a very long way in treating babies with Down syndrome and in recognizing their great potential. There are some, however, who may cling to stereotypes and outdated information. Be sure you pick a doctor who is current in both knowledge and attitude. Switch doctors if you find your doctor has beliefs and biases that make you uncomfortable. If your doctor expresses low expectations for your child, switch doctors; you do not have to tolerate this. Do not hesitate to get second opinions, or third opinions if you feel they are necessary.

Don't Let the Paperwork Bury You. Being sick today is not what it used to be. To parents, it must seem there is a sea of forms to fill out, and a sea of bills and statements to decipher. Complex insurance forms are often very difficult, as well as time-consuming, to sort out—and they usually descend upon you right when you are trying to deal with a medical problem. Do not feel pressured to stay on top of your forms. There are no more stressful times for you and your child than when your child is ill. Although it is not advisable to be late on medical bills, be sure to take time for your child *and for yourself* before attacking that mountain of bills. If possible, wait until after your child's treatment is over—at least until it is less intense. Take some time to breathe, *then* tackle the pile of papers. Also, do not be afraid to call your doctor or your insurance company with questions. They are there to help *you.*

Keep a Notebook. Because there are so many specialists that you and your child might need to see, it may be very helpful to keep a notebook. List questions and addresses and telephone numbers, and take notes on your consultations and meetings. This notebook can also be used to keep a record of your written observations of your child, along with tests and evaluations.

One last suggestion: you may be entitled to up to twelve weeks of unpaid leave from your job to help care for a serious medical need of your child with Down syndrome. The "Family and Medical Leave Act of 1993" requires employers of 50 or more people to allow their employees unpaid leave without the risk of job loss. You may want to check into this law and discuss it with your employer if you need extra time away from work to deal with your child's medical needs.

Conclusion

After reading this chapter you may think that babies with Down syndrome are always sick and in need of medical care. That is simply not the case. Babies with Down syndrome generally enjoy good health. Problems can come up, but there are effective treatments for virtually every one of them. And most children do not have all of the problems discussed in this chapter.

In recent decades, medical science has come a long way in helping children with Down syndrome lead more healthy and vigorous lives. Problems that not too long ago meant premature death are now treatable. Problems that hindered development and prevented children from reaching their full developmental potential now pose far less serious threats. With better overall health, improved medical care, and close monitoring by parents and professionals, there is every reason to expect your child with Down syndrome to lead a full and healthy life.

References

Eyman, R.K., Call, T.I., White, J.F. "Life Expectancy of Persons with Down Syndrome." *American Journal of Mental Retardation.* Vol. 95, 1991, 603–612.

Spicer, R.L. "Cardiovascular Disease in Down Syndrome." *Pediatric Clinics of North America.* Vol. 31, no. 6, 1984, 1331–1343.

Pueschel, S.M. "Clinical aspects of Down Syndrome From Infancy to Adulthood." *A.J.Med.Genet.* Vol. 7, 1990, 52–56.

Caputo, A.R., Wagner, R.S., Reynolds, D.R., Guo, S., Goel, A.K. "Down Syndrome: Clinical Review of Ocular Features." *Clinical Pediatrics.* Vol. 28, 1989, 355–358.

Diamond, L.S., Lynne, D., Sigman, B. "Disorders in Patients with Down Syndrome." *Orthopedic Clinics of North America.* Vol. 12, No. 1, 1981, 57–71.

Carey, J.C. "Health Supervision and Anticipatory Guidance For Children With Genetic Disorders." *Pediatric Clinics Of North America.* Vol. 39, 1992, 25–53.

Down Syndrome Preventive Medical Check List (1994). National Down Syndrome Congress.

Capone, G.T. "Molecular Advances Toward Understanding Down Syndrome." *Down Syndrome Papers and Abstracts for Professionals.*, Vol. 15, 1992, 1–3.

Shapiro, B. "Normal and Abnormal Development: Down Syndrome." In Batshaw M.L., Perret Y.M. (eds), *Children With Disabilities: A Medical Primer.* Baltimore: Paul H. Brookes Publishing Co. 1992, 272–278.

Zigman, W.B., Schupf, N., Lubin, R., Silverman, W. "Premature Regression of Adults with Down Syndrome." *American Journal of Mental Deficiency.* Vol. 92, 1987, 161–168.

Pueschel, S.M. "The Child with Down Syndrome." In Levine, Carey, Crocker, & Gross. *Developmental Behavioral Pediatrics.* Philadelphia: W.B. Saunders Co. 1983, 353–362.

Parent Statements

We have been quite pleased with the medical attention he has gotten. The children's hospital here has been very understanding; they seem to be assertive about their medical practice. You know, they would make sure that he got tests for his heart and all the things that could happen that we wouldn't have known about. They made sure that he had tests and they followed up.

When we found out she had a heart defect, it almost didn't matter. That's really awful to say, but we almost couldn't have felt worse. We had just found out she had Down syndrome, and we felt the heart thing was something we could take care of. We felt we could manage it better.

We feel it's extremely important to get vision and hearing check-ups. You need to know there is a problem to help the problem. Many children with Down syndrome speak later than other children and you need to give them every chance to speak and to hear what you're saying. It is the same thing with vision.

I think physicians have a responsibility to give you all the options and let you make the decisions. But I don't think anyone ever suggested that she not have her heart surgery. Even with her failing to thrive and with her not gaining weight and doing absolutely awful, it was never recommended that we give up in any way.

I can't understand *not* allowing life-saving surgery. I was shocked once when a doctor actually gave me the option of not authorizing emergency abdominal surgery. Mike deserves the same chance to live his life as any other child. For heaven's sake, he's my child.

I've always felt that it's open season on Mike. I mean the kid's been x-rayed a lot. He has had heart problems and he had abdominal surgery. They are really quick to order medical procedures and tests they might not otherwise order.

Our little boy has hypothyroidism. We were so glad it was diagnosed early because we were able to start medication immediately. Otherwise, he'd have other problems on top of Down syndrome. But we caught it early enough, and now we just give him medicine once a day.

She had no colds, no pneumonia, no nothing, until this year, until she was three. The doctor feels it was not related to having Down syndrome; it was just a bad year. She had high exposure to many children this year, because she was in nursery school.

When Hope was four months old, she had a lot of fluid in her ears. She didn't act as if her ears hurt, though, and didn't show any noticeable (to us) signs of hearing loss. Fortunately, our geneticist had recommended that we have her hearing tested at around this age. The test detected a moderate hearing loss in one ear, so we took her to an ear, nose, and throat specialist. This doctor discovered that Hope had fluid in both ears. After three or four months, the fluid was still there, so the doctor recommended surgically inserting tubes in her eardrums to drain the fluid and equalize the pressure in her ears. After the surgery, Hope's hearing was normal, and has remained normal for a year now. Just as importantly, her speech is developing really well, which I doubt would be the case if we hadn't identified and fixed her hearing problem so early.

＊ ＾ ＊ ＾ ＊ ＾ ＊ ＾ ＊

Mike has a good dose of ADHD in addition to Down syndrome (it seems to run in my family). He's been evaluated and prescribed Ritalin. I know that Ritalin is somewhat controversial, but I have to say that we notice significant differences in Mike's behavior. When he is on Ritalin, he is much more "available" for learning—he can sit still, pay attention, and keep focused long enough to learn something. Before, it was very hard for him. So I figure, at least for Mike, why not make learning as easy for him as we can—it is already hard enough.

＊ ＾ ＊ ＾ ＊ ＾ ＊ ＾ ＊

I think hearing should be checked in the same way that people vote in Chicago—early and often. Communication is so important for children with Down syndrome, and hearing is essential for the development of communication skills. Ear infections and fluid can change your child's hearing very quickly, and can really slow, or even reverse, progress she has made in learning to communicate. Our son has a mild hearing loss and wears hearing aids. Sure, they are a bother and expensive, but I would never take the chance of robbing him of something essential to his learning to communicate.

The medical professionals have been very thorough. Sometimes it has caused him too much pain for the end result. It's a function of his having Down syndrome and therefore he has to suffer being probed a bit more because he has higher chances of this or that. Now he just breaks into hysterical sobs whenever he sees a doctor.

I spoke to a parent not long ago who had just given birth to a baby with Down syndrome. That woman had five different doctors. She had a two-day-old baby, and they all had something different to say. None of them were conferring with the others. She was already the team leader and didn't know enough to lead the team. It was just overwhelming for her.

Certain things worked well for us in dealing with the doctors. We ask a lot of questions, and don't let them get away with not answering or with putting things in language we can't understand. We're paying them to help our child and we need to understand what they're saying. People shouldn't be embarrassed to not understand.

I wanted somebody who, even if they didn't know, would help me find out. I think an important function of a pediatrician is to coordinate your child's care. Some programs do this for your child, but many do not. The pediatrician needs to be aware of what speech is doing, what OT is doing, what physical therapy is doing, what cognitive is doing, what the geneticist is doing, what the ophthalmologist is doing, what the audiologist is doing. We found a pediatrician who reads everything he gets about Laurie, calls me if something doesn't jibe, and really is a coordinator.

We were sort of disappointed in our regular pediatrician. After seeing Josh about four times, he said, "Are you having any special therapy for this boy?" He was just beginning to show signs of a speech delay, and I think the doctor didn't even remember that we were doing everything we could. This pediatrician was strictly inoculations and regular check-ups. He really wasn't prepared to deal with Down syndrome at all.

Most doctors don't know "boo" about Down syndrome. But they can't admit it. So it's very frustrating to deal with a doctor when you know more than they do about the special needs of your child.

If the experience is not helpful to you, change it. We had a pediatrician who kept saying "these children," patted me on the head, and told me not to worry, that this is what life was going to be like and I might as well get used to it. But I decided that I wanted to do everything I could and I wasn't getting the impression that this doctor was giving me everything I could do. I had a lot of guilt because I always tend to think a doctor is right— he's the expert. It took me about a month before it dawned on me to go exploring for someone who would be positive.

Sometimes it takes courage to change. Maybe the pediatrician that you have is the one the whole family uses, but doesn't have a clue about dealing with the special problems of kids with disabilities. Maybe the person that you picked out isn't suitable.

You have to make changes. Never put any of these other considerations, or your own uneasiness about terminating people's services, before the best interests of your child.

~ ~ ~ ~ ~ ~ ~ ~ ~ ~

Insurance is a major concern. Persistence can have rewards and if the first time you don't succeed in getting payment for a particular service, keep trying. It could be because the person at that level didn't understand. Or maybe the services are not covered for a particular diagnosis but if you get another diagnosis that really is the same thing but just said in a different way, the policy will cover it. Or if that doesn't work, maybe there is someone else at the next level who has the authority to take it on appeal. Just keep at it. Save all your copies and keep submitting all your documents. Keep going higher and higher up, because once you concede that something is not covered there's no going back. They expect you to give up, but you might get lucky. You may get somebody in the chain of command who will make a reverse decision or you may be perfectly within your rights to expect coverage for a particular service.

Four

~~~~~~~~

The Daily Care
of Your Baby

Joan Burggraf Riley, R.N., M.S.N.*
and Elliot Gersh, M.D.**

Many parents of babies with Down syndrome feel that the daily care of their child is very similar to the care of other children. Perhaps for this reason there is very little written about the daily care of children with Down syndrome. However, because your baby may be different from other children in some ways, her daily care will sometimes require special knowledge and effort. This chapter explores those areas of daily care that are unique to babies with Down syndrome.

A tremendous amount has been written about child care in general. Eating, sleeping, bathing, and diapering are extensively covered in hundreds of baby care books. These general baby care books can be helpful, but their advice must be adapted to your child's special needs. Supplement these books with this chapter's information.

Routine activities—eating, bathing, and diapering—are major events in a baby's or toddler's day. You can tailor your baby's activities to enhance her development simply by being aware of

---

* Joan Burggraf Riley, is a Registered Nurse and a Clinical Instructor at the Georgetown University School of Nursing in Washington, D.C.

** Elliot Gersh, M.D. is a developmental pediatrician at the Georgetown University Child Development Center in Washington, D.C.

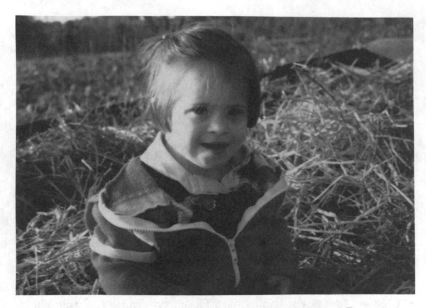

your child's development as you go through each day. But remember: Babies with Down syndrome are babies first and foremost. Care for her as you would any other baby. Follow your instincts, but in those areas where your baby has special needs, use the information in this chapter to deal with those needs effectively.

Routine and Discipline

One of the most important aspects of your baby's daily care is to set a routine. A routine allows your baby to learn what to expect in her daily activities. A routine sets an order to her day, and makes her feel safe. Routine within each daily activity provides security and teaches your baby about the activity. For example, a bedtime routine of a bath and a story book teaches her about how bedtime happens. Routine will later allow your child to participate in her other daily activities.

Routines differ for each family because of each family member's schedule and because of each baby's schedule. For example, some families give their babies a bath in the evening in order to help them calm down and relax, while other families give their babies baths in the morning because their babies get very excited splashing around and playing in the water. In either case, the consistency of your routine will benefit both you and your baby.

You may also need to reassess your family style in light of your baby's particular needs. Limit-setting and consistency—discipline in general—are important for any child. But for a baby with Down syndrome you may need to be more deliberate about it. Families with a child with Down syndrome report that they find it necessary to verbalize rules other children in their family take for granted. For example, if your family dinnertime routine is very casual, you may have to adjust your methods to your child's special needs. On the other hand, if your family routine tends to be highly structured, you might have to allow for more flexibility. Most likely, your particular style is just fine. Just remember that it is important to be aware of how your daily activities, style, and expectations can affect your baby's development. Your goal in providing routine and structure is to create an environment in which your child will have trust in the people and things in her life. Other children may manage to get along fine without this deliberate level of care, but if you optimize your special baby's environment, you will help her reach her full potential.

Don't let your baby's Down syndrome spoil her. Discipline and routine are just as important to her as to any other baby. You will be surprised at how clever she is at manipulating you. Your child will have to learn how to behave, and you won't be doing her a favor if you fail to enforce the do's and do-not's.

You want your child to be an active participant in her community. Appropriate behavior is essential for her to be included in peer groups, social settings, and the community at large, and appropriate behavior is a *learned* skill. If you allow your child to throw food at home or to hit her brother or sister, you cannot expect her to know that these behaviors are unacceptable. Simple, consistent, and clear directions will be the most helpful tools you can use to establish discipline guidelines for your child. As your child gets into the preschool and school-age years, teach

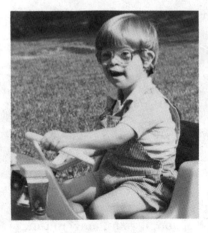

her to observe how her peer group is behaving and to model her own behavior after theirs.

Eating

From birth onward, mealtime is one of the most important times parents spend with their child. Babies are usually alert and attentive while they are eating, and mealtime can be an enjoyable time for all family members to get together. As your child grows, she will enjoy being with the rest of her family, participating in the discussion about everyone's daily activities.

Children with Down syndrome have to learn feeding skills, and this process requires time and patience. It takes practice for your baby to learn to feed herself, and—like other children—there will be plenty of messes. You have to be ready to wipe up spills and clean up faces and hands. But rest assured, all babies with Down syndrome learn to feed themselves.

Breast or Bottle Feeding

Babies with Down syndrome can breast or bottle feed like other children, but may need a little extra help. It may be harder at first for them to feed in a coordinated way, but most learn quickly to be good breast or bottle feeders. If you understand your baby's potential feeding problems and how to overcome them, feeding can become a special time for both of you.

Whether you are breastfeeding or bottle feeding your baby, regular checkups with her health care provider are essential to monitor her nutritional health. This can be particularly important because possible medical problems with her heart and her low muscle tone can result in a weak suck. If she breastfeeds, consult your health care provider for the name and phone number of a lactation consultant to provide expert guidance as you learn the mechanics of breastfeeding. Some areas have organizations where women volunteer to provide support and guidance to new mothers based on their personal experience.

Babies and children with Down syndrome sometimes have physical characteristics that affect how they eat. Your child's mouth may be smaller, allowing her tongue to protrude. The muscles of her lips, tongue, and cheeks may not move in a coordinated fashion due to low muscle tone. Consequently, your baby with Down syndrome may have more difficulty getting a tight seal on a nipple. She may have a weaker suck, and later may have more difficulty moving food around in her mouth as she chews. As you work with your baby's teacher or therapist, you will be amazed at how complex the act of eating can be and how it is affected by your baby's development.

Some babies require special techniques to strengthen eating skills if their oral motor development is not normal. These techniques stimulate some of the natural patterns your child has for sucking, rooting, and swallowing. Frequently, parents need instruction from someone familiar with these techniques— either your child's therapist or teacher. In general, it is a good idea to have a speech therapist check your baby's eating patterns and oral motor skills to help you provide the best feeding stimulation. Remember, these techniques require time and practice. To stimulate your baby's natural rooting and sucking mechanisms, you can rub her cheeks toward the mouth with your hand or a soft cloth. This should make her pucker. The best time to do this is just before mealtime to stimulate her oral reflexes. You should also encourage her to suck on her hand, fist, or fingers. These normal hand-to-mouth activities will help her develop good oral patterns.

Pacifiers can also help strengthen your baby's suck. You can choose from a wide variety of shapes, sizes, and materials. Your baby may respond more positively to one than another, so be ready for some experimenting. The pacifier helps strengthen oral motor control and can help soothe your baby if she is upset. But remember that, just like other babies, your child may not want or need to use a pacifier.

You can also use the nipple of the breast or the bottle to stimulate your baby's rooting and sucking reflexes. Gentle pressure on her cheeks or lips will get her to turn her head toward the nipple. Your baby will need good lip closure on the nipple, and you can help her by holding her in a flexed position. This position is tight in your arms with your baby's knees and arms held snug into her trunk. Good lip closure is also helped by rubbing her cheeks toward her lips, and rubbing upward from her chin and downward from her nose toward her lips. These actions help your baby to be more organized and focused on her feeding.

If you choose to bottle feed your baby, there is quite a wide variety of commercial nipples available. Your baby may prefer one commercial nipple to another. In choosing a commercial nipple, you should check to see that there is a nice, even flow of milk. There is also a wide variety of bottles. For a child with a weak suck it may be helpful to use a soft plastic bottle or disposable plastic bag. Either of these will allow you to apply gentle pressure on the bottle or bag to help milk flow out evenly. Once you choose a particular nipple, use only that same style for all bottle feeding. Avoid switching nipple styles. Each different nipple style requires a slightly different suck. Switching around will not allow your baby to learn and master a particular suck pattern and will frustrate and confuse her.

Babies need good support to eat comfortably and efficiently. Low muscle tone makes it more difficult for your baby to hold herself in a good position, which is crucial to proper sucking and swallowing. At first the mother or father must provide good support for their baby. Obviously, the type of support depends on your baby's age and developmental level. When they are tiny, babies should be held in a semi-upright position with good head support, with the head tilted slightly forward. A newborn should be cradled snugly and securely in your arms with her legs supported in your lap.

There are two ways to arrange your baby's mealtimes: you can establish a schedule or you can feed her on demand. With demand feeding you offer your baby food when she shows she is hungry and ready to eat. Scheduled feeding means that you set a routine, usually feeding your baby at three- to four-hour intervals. Babies with Down syndrome generally do best when they are fed on demand. Learn to recognize your baby's signs that she is hungry. Many babies whine or get fidgety before they cry to express hunger. If your baby has difficulty eating, mealtime will go more smoothly when she is hungry and ready to eat. Any baby will concentrate better when awake, alert, and giving

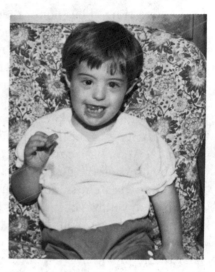

signs that she is hungry, such as lip-smacking, hand-to-mouth activity, restlessness, fussing, rooting, sticking out her tongue, or crying.

Some babies with Down syndrome tend to sleep through what should be their mealtime. Your health care provider may suggest you wake up your baby on a schedule during the day in order to give her adequate feedings and allow her longer sleeping periods at night. Monitor your baby's feeding to make sure she is getting enough nutrition and consult with her health care provider.

Introducing Solid Foods

Your baby can be introduced to solid foods at the same age as other children. This usually occurs from four to six months of age, but some parents wait as long as a year. It is generally recommended that babies with Down syndrome be introduced to solid foods by six months of age. Eating solid foods helps develop a number of important skills, including fine motor skills and sensory awareness in the mouth. More importantly, babies with Down syndrome can be especially sensitive to differing textures; if this happens, they may balk at trying different foods. Some babies with Down syndrome gag or swallow too much food at one time. The sooner they can work through this, the better. Check with your baby's health care provider or teacher to determine when your child is ready to start eating solid food. And remember that the introduction of solid foods does not substitute for nutrition received through breast or formula feedings.

When you do introduce new foods, give your baby a choice of either commercially prepared, pureed baby foods, or foods pureed at home. Both options are fine. Commercial baby food companies now emphasize nutrition in the preparation of their foods by limiting the amount of added salt and sugar. The order in which foods are introduced varies, but many people first offer cereal, then yellow vegetables, green vegetables, and fruit, with meats and fish last. Your baby may not like all these foods, but what baby does? Just strive for a balanced diet. Consult your health care provider to establish nutritional guidelines for your baby.

Give your baby small amounts of new food each day for several days to see that she can tolerate it. Babies will often push food out of their mouth with their tongues. When this happens, you can try putting a small amount of food onto the middle part of her tongue with some downward pressure from the spoon. You can also try applying some gentle pressure on her upper and lower lips to keep her mouth closed around the food.

As babies gain control over solids, they start finger feeding, a very important and enjoyable activity for them. Finger feeding provides babies with independence as well as with another way to explore their environment. In addition, finger feeding develops sensory awareness and fine motor control.

Finger feeding is an extension of the hand-to-mouth activity begun at a very early age. You should offer your baby a large variety of finger foods. Sticky foods are good for children who have not yet developed a good grasp with their fingers. Try cottage cheese, yogurt, or pudding so your baby can dip her fingers into the food and bring it to her mouth. Later on, when your baby develops a better grasp, she can start reaching for small bits of food like Cheerios, cooked pasta, cooked vegetables, and fruits.

When your baby starts to use her own spoon, you will have to try some of the different sizes and shapes available. Often conventional adult spoons are difficult for a baby to use in the beginning; she will have more success if the spoon is easier to hold and place in her mouth. You can buy baby spoons with flatter bowls and wider grips. Some have small holes in the bowl that help keep the food sitting on the spoon until your baby places it in her mouth. Again, it is a good idea to have a therapist check the way your baby takes the food from the spoon and the way she holds and moves the spoon.

Proper posture and support are as crucial for eating as they are for breast or bottle feeding. How your baby sits affects how well she can manipulate food and hold a spoon. Your child should be fed in a high chair with her feet well supported, her trunk secure, and the height of the table at elbow level. Some children benefit from foam supports in their high chair to keep them in a proper position before they can easily do it themselves. You should ask your child's teacher or therapist whether your child needs the extra support and where she needs it.

Mealtimes with your child will be noisy and hectic; they can also be enjoyable. Like all children, your child may often wear more food than she eats. What can you do to prevent mealtimes from becoming too chaotic?

First, consistent discipline is essential. Behavior such as standing on a chair should be discouraged. Set standards for all your children and hold them to it. But remember, mealtimes are excellent opportunities to work on development, language, and self-help skills. Strike a balance and strive for enjoyable mealtimes, knowing that they can be both rewarding and frustrating.

Drinking from a Cup

How soon your child makes the transition from breast or bottle feeding to cup drinking depends on your child's ability to reach, grasp, and control a cup. By the time your baby is ready to drink from a cup she already has taken an active role in holding her bottle and can bring it to her mouth. For good cup drinking, your baby has to be able to sip from the cup rather than suck. This can be encouraged initially by having your baby take liquids from a cup with a wide lip or a cup with a lid that allows small amounts of liquid to pass through holes in the lid. Cups with spouts are not a good idea because they promote sucking.

While your baby drinks, pay close attention to make sure she is not resting the cup on her tongue instead of on her lower lip. Babies are tempted to do this because it is easier to hold the cup still with the tongue than with the lower lip. This is particularly true if your child is used to sticking her tongue out. This habit is difficult to break when your child is older, so it is a good idea to discourage it early. Giving gentle support under the chin can enable your child to hold the cup in the right position without using her tongue. Your teacher or therapist can be very helpful in teaching your child to drink correctly from a cup.

Weight Gain

Some babies with Down syndrome have difficulty gaining weight. This is generally a problem among children who have a congenital heart defect. This is usually a concern during the first year of life. These babies should be monitored by their cardiologist and health care provider. Special diets and other medical treatment can be prescribed to improve weight gain.

Your child should have her growth monitored, using a special growth chart for children with Down syndrome. Figure 1 shows two growth charts with the range of growth for girls and boys with Down syndrome. Children with Down syndrome have a slower rate of growth than other children. The important thing is to maintain balance between weight gain and growth in height. Never settle for the outdated stereotype of the fat and inactive child with Down syndrome.

Parents of a child with Down syndrome need to pay particular attention to their child's weight gain. Studies of children with Down syndrome have found that approximately 30 percent develop obesity. This obesity is usually caused by a combination of overeating and inactivity. An additional factor is that children are frequently rewarded for activities with sweets and high calorie foods. Be aware that early dietary habits and preferences can

Figure 1. Growth Charts for Boys and Girls with Down Syndrome

Down Syndrome-Physical Growth, Males, 0–36 Months

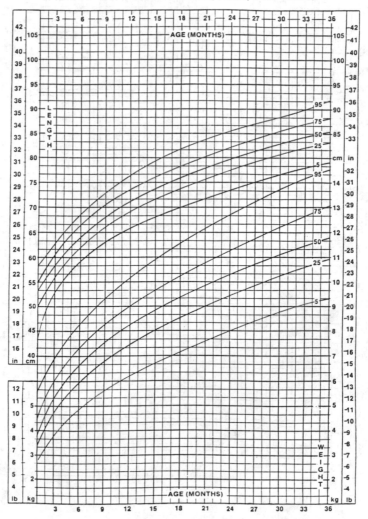

Height and weight for males with Down syndrome birth to 36 months of age. Data collected at the Developmental Evaluation Clinic of the Children's Hospital Boston, The Child Development Center of Rhode Island Hospital and the Clinical Genetics Service of the Children's Hospital of Philadelphia. Copyright, C.E. Cronk, A.C. Crocker, S.M. Pueschel and E. Zachai, 1986. Cronk CE: *Pediatrics* 61:564, 1978; Cronk CE et al: *Pediatrics* 81:102, 1988.

Down Syndrome-Physical Growth, Males, 2–18 Years

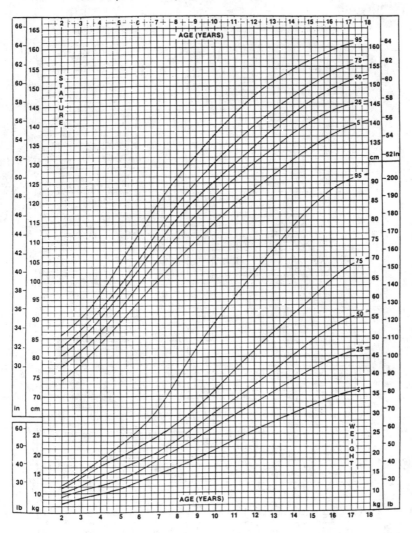

Height and weight for males with Down syndrome 2 to 18 years of age.
(Cronk, CE et al: *Pediatrics* 81:102, 1988.)

Down Syndrome-Physical Growth, Females, 0–36 Months

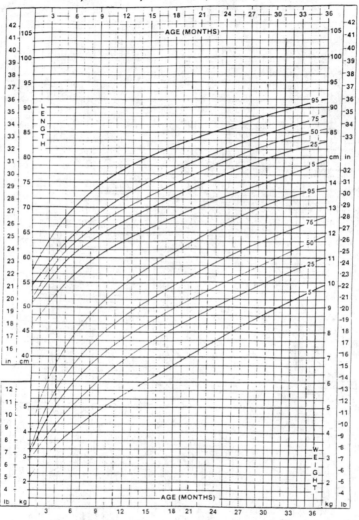

Height and weight for females with Down syndrome, birth to 36 months of age. (Cronk, CE et al: *Pediatrics* 81: 102, 1988.)

Down Syndrome-Physical Growth, Females, 2–18 Years

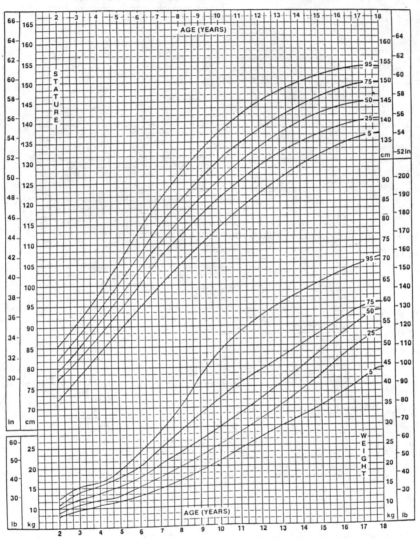

Height and weight for females with Down syndrome 2 to 18 years of age.
(Cronk, CE et al: *Pediatrics* 81:102, 1988.)

influence life long nutrition. Consult your child's health care provider with your concerns and questions about your baby's weight gain. As your baby grows, continue to have periodic discussions about your child's unique nutritional needs to prevent obesity.

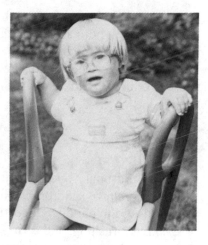

Constipation

Many children with Down syndrome have difficulty with constipation. Constipation is defined as an intestinal dysfunction in which it is difficult or painful to have bowel movements. Parents have differing expectations about their babies' stooling. What infants eat influences their stooling. For example, breast fed babies may have 4 to 6 stools per day, while bottle fed babies may have 1 to 3 stools per day. The frequency and consistency of your baby's bowel movements and your concerns should be discussed with your health care provider.

The difficulty your baby with Down syndrome has with constipation may be due to low muscle tone, which makes it more difficult for her to develop a good push for a bowel movement. There are helpful steps you can take. First, control your child's diet. It is important to have a good balance of whole grain cereals, vegetables, fruits, and plenty of liquids. This helps digestion and minimizes constipation. Second, constipation generally responds to increasing fluid intake. Constipation often becomes a problem for toddlers when their fluid intake decreases and they begin to eat more solid foods. Third, if you notice your child struggling during bowel movements, try flexing her legs up to her abdomen. This puts pressure on the belly and helps your child to push.

The treatment of constipation must be tailored to each individual child. You should consult with your child's health care provider about constipation problems. He or she can provide treatment and monitor this problem to meet your child's individual needs. There are numerous over-the-counter remedies for constipation which should never be given to your child without the advice of your child's health care provider. Some of these products could be dangerous for infants and young children.

Hygiene

Good personal hygiene habits are important for children and adults with Down syndrome. The foundation for good hygiene is established in childhood; getting your child into the pattern of washing, brushing, and caring for herself is a critical skill for the future. This section reviews some of the basics of daily care for your child.

Bathing and Skin Care

Many parents bathe their children daily, but this may not be necessary as long as you keep your child's diaper area and face and mouth clean. While your child is a newborn, you can give her sponge baths using a soft cloth. After her umbilical stump falls off, you can bathe her in a wash bowl, sink, or baby bathtub. And, when she is older and you feel more secure, she can be bathed in a tub. There are many safety devices available commercially for use when bathing your baby. None of these is essential and some devices can be dangerous because they can provide false confidence that your baby is safe in the bathtub. Nothing replaces the safety of your hands and eyes on your baby during bath time.

Children with Down syndrome have a tendency to develop dry skin, with areas of rough, red, flaky, or irritated patches on the legs, buttocks, arms, hands, and feet. To prevent and control this, it is important to develop a good skin care routine. You should use moisturizing soaps (Basis, Dove, Caress, Tone), and apply lotion (Eucerin, Nivea, Aquaphor) immediately after bathing while the skin is still moist. What the lotion does is to lock in the moisture the skin absorbed when bathing. Applying lotion to dry skin is not very effective. Apply lotion more than once a day, particularly on the hands and face after mealtime wiping. If the problem persists, consult your health care provider. He or she can prescribe more potent skin lotions or suggest other ways to treat dry skin.

Parents often ask about the scalp, which can become crusted and flaky. This "cradle cap" is quite common in the early months of your baby's life and is part of the scalp's normal way of shedding dead skin cells. The best treatment is to rub petroleum jelly into the scalp to soften crusts 20 to 30 minutes prior to shampooing. Shampoo your baby's hair daily with baby shampoo. Gently brush the scalp with a soft brush during bathing to remove the dead skin. It is all right to gently wash over "soft spots." Keep the shampoo out of your baby's eyes. Continue daily shampooing for several days after the cradle cap disappears. Then shampoo at least weekly thereafter.

It is important to keep the diaper area clean. Wash the skin with plain water with each diaper change to prevent diaper rash. It may be helpful to routinely use a lubricant such as petroleum jelly, Desitin, or other baby diaper skin care product to protect the skin from dryness and irritation. Do not use cornstarch as it can encourage the growth of bacteria and fungi.

It is possible your child's skin is sensitive to the brand of diaper you are using. If you suspect sensitivity switch to another brand of diaper. Always fold the plastic top of the diaper *away* from the body. The best treatment of diaper rash is prevention. If your baby develops a rash that is not clearing up with these prevention techniques, consult your health care provider.

Diapering can be an excellent time to incorporate developmental activities into your baby's routine. It is an opportunity for talking to your baby while making eye contact. Playful touching at this time can provide helpful stimulation for your baby. At the very least, diapering is a good time to be sociable, to talk to your baby, to stroke her body, and to help her move her arms and legs. Your baby's teacher or therapist may also have some good ideas on positions and movements during diapering.

Toilet Training

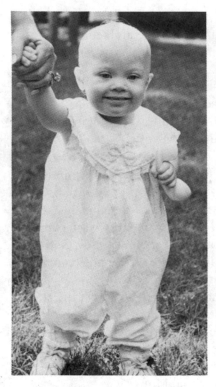

Many children with Down syndrome do not become toilet trained during the first three years of life, although there is a wide range of accomplishments in this area. As with other children, toilet training can be quite a struggle, but your child *will* become toilet trained.

Many books and pamphlets have been published to help parents toilet train their children. As your child grows, she will start to become aware of her bodily functions. At that point, she will need to know how to ask to go to the bathroom. Toilet training requires many areas of development to come together at once—such as communication, muscle control, and awareness of bodily functions. Look for signs or cues that your child is aware that she has a wet diaper or has had a bowel movement, such as showing discomfort and asking to have her diaper changed. These signs let you know that your child is aware of her toileting needs. Have a potty chair available when she is ready.

Some authorities on toilet training advocate gradually guiding a child to using the toilet. Other authorities suggest waiting for the child to show readiness or awareness of toileting needs. Be careful not to place pressure on your child to toilet train. Avoid overly praising her for success on the toilet; praise should be consistent with the praise given for her other accomplishments. It is important to remember that this is only one of the many tasks your child is attempting to master at one time and to understand her frequent lapses.

We do not include specific techniques in toilet training in this chapter. When your child reaches that stage, refer to the books in the Reading List, and if necessary, seek the help of your baby's teachers, therapists, and health care providers.

Eyes

Like other children, babies with Down syndrome sometimes develop blockages in a tear duct, resulting in increased tearing or crusting of the eye. In some children this corrects itself, while in others it may require medical treatment. To help avoid blocked tear ducts, you can clean your baby's eyelids by wiping gently from the inner corner outward toward the ear. This can be done with a clean moist washcloth or cotton ball.

Ears

Barring ear infections (discussed in Chapter 3), your baby's ears can receive normal care. Ear wax builds up naturally in the ears and works its way out. Some children with Down syndrome require ear cleaning on a routine basis. Their ears are not able to cleanse themselves and ear wax builds up over time. Ear wax buildup can decrease hearing and hinder language development. Your child's health care provider can look in your child's ears to determine if this is a problem for your child. Therefore, there is no need to insert *any* object into the ear canal. You just need to clean the outer ear and the area behind the ear by gently washing and drying.

Nose

Some children with Down syndrome have more frequent runny noses and thickened secretions due to smaller nasal passages. Usually, the use of a cool mist humidifier in your baby's room is recommended. This will help loosen secretions and make it easier for your baby to breathe.

To clean the outside of the nose, wipe it with a warm, moistened cloth such as a diaper or soft cotton washcloth. Occasionally, nose secretions become dry and crusted around the outside of the nose. You can remove these gently with the use of a lotion or a cream. Try not to irritate the nose further by frequent wiping. Petroleum jelly or lotion will also ease the irritation. If the inside of your baby's nose becomes dry and crusty, ask your health care provider about saline nose drops. Nasal aspirators do not work well and may cause irritation.

Teeth

As with any child, it is important to instill good habits of dental care at an early age. This benefits your child in a number of ways. First, if your baby breathes with her mouth open much of the time, there can be an extra build-up of tartar in her mouth. Second, brushing helps stimulate a number of developmental skills—from getting used to sensory stimulation all around the mouth, to practicing sound production in the mirror, to learning how to handle the toothbrush by herself. To avoid dental problems later, good oral hygiene is essential now.

The care of your child's teeth is not different from other children. Cleaning of the teeth should begin as soon as teeth erupt. Wipe your baby's first teeth with gauze before bedtime each night. A soft toothbrush can be used as early as your child can tolerate it. Once your child is two to three years old she should brush her own teeth twice a day to encourage good hygiene habits, but at bedtime you should complete the toothbrushing. Most children lack the manual dexterity to brush satisfactorily until they are about six years old.

Two years old is the age recommended by the Academy of Pediatric Dentistry for your child's first dental appointment. This examination will reveal your child's tooth eruption pattern and will provide an opportunity for oral hygiene instruction. By the time your child is three years of age, she will be familiar with the dental office and staff, and will be able to participate in the dental exam, cleaning, and fluoride treatment.

Holding Your Baby

It is very important to be conscious of how your baby positions herself and how she moves. In addition to low muscle tone, babies with Down syndrome often have very loose joints. This allows their limbs to settle into positions that might lead to problems when they start to sit, crawl, and walk. Many parents find it helpful to consult a physical therapist soon after birth to ask about positioning. There are simple changes you can make in the way you might instinctively hold your baby, changes that would stabilize her joints and help support her better. For example, it helps to hold your baby so that her legs are together, rather than wrapped around your hips.

Early patterns of movement can influence later development and are crucial to future social acceptance and self-esteem. Children with Down syndrome who move normally can do more of the things other children can do, like climb, run, and play. Good motor development will improve your child's posture, mobility, coordination, and endurance. How you hold your baby will help her in these areas later in life. Consult with your baby's health care provider and teachers for suggestions about holding your child. Remember, good development is the product of careful attention to a number of small details.

All of this concern about how you hold your child may sound intimidating. Unless your baby has a particular medical problem, however, don't handle her as though she were made of glass. She will love "roughhousing" and active play, just as other children do. Not only is this activity good for sensory stimulation, but it sends to your baby and your other children the message that you intend to treat her as an equal member of the family. If you set this example, family and friends will follow your lead.

Exercise

Exercise is critical to children with Down syndrome. It can break the vicious cycle of low muscle tone leading to inactivity, inactivity leading to obesity, obesity leading to more inactivity, and so on and so on. Because low muscle tone requires your baby to work harder to move, you need to take an active role in monitoring her movements, designing a good exercise program, and motivating her to move around.

A physical therapist, teacher, and selected books can get you and your baby started on an exercise program. Your baby's teacher can also make sure that your baby's exercise actually aids development. Strengthening muscles, improving coordination, and learning balance all can help tremendously in many areas of development.

Sleep and Rest

Newborns do not have predictable sleep patterns. They often sleep most of the time and wake primarily to eat. Of course, each child is different, but generally newborns with Down syndrome have typical sleep patterns. As your child grows, the periods of wakefulness and sleep both increase. By two to three months of age, your baby's sleep becomes more organized, and a regular pattern develops.

Parents learn early to interpret their baby's cues for sleep as well as for hunger and attention. Your baby will express her needs for each of these with different cries, movements, and vocalizations. You will come to know when it is time for your baby to sleep—hopefully when *you* want to sleep—and when it is time to be awake. Once asleep, your baby's level of sleep varies, and she frequently will make noises, twitch, and move. These are all normal signs of sleep.

As in all daily care activities, routine is important. Many parents complain that their children won't sleep through the night, or won't settle down without being held or without being allowed to sleep in Mom and Dad's bed. Don't assume your child needs comforting any more or less because she has Down syndrome. She will be just as quick as any other child to manipulate you in your attempts to settle her down for the night. A regular sleep and bedtime routine consistently enforced may help to avoid these problems. For example, if your child gets in the pattern of selecting a favorite toy to sleep with and listens to a book or story at bedtime, she will learn to associate these activities with going to bed.

Child Care

Any caring and careful person with whom you feel comfortable can baby-sit your baby. If your baby has seizures or other serious medical problems, a babysitter with special training should be used. Otherwise, no special training is required. Of course, you will need to spend some time showing the babysitter how your baby eats, sleeps, or plays, but you would do this for any child. The important thing to remember is that it is good for *everyone* if you get a babysitter once in a while. You need to take some time for yourself, and your baby needs to learn to deal with people other than family members.

It is often difficult for new parents to leave their baby with Down syndrome with a babysitter. This is especially true if your child has medical problems. The constant fear that an emergency will arise when you are out can trap you at home unnecessarily, depriving you of valuable opportunities for enjoyment. With a competent babysitter, however, this problem can be easily avoided.

If you prefer a trained baby sitter, contact your local chapter of The Arc (formerly called the Association for Retarded Citizens), your local Down syndrome parents support group, or the special education department of your local college or university. They may have a list of sitters in your area who specialize in child care for children with special needs. Another idea is to start a pool of parents (especially other parents of children with Down syndrome) who are willing to trade babysitting with you.

Selecting a Health Care Provider

Most health care providers are well equipped to care for a child with Down syndrome. In recent years, there has been a trend toward community-based care of children with disabilities, including children with Down syndrome. This means that regular pediatricians, family practitioners, and nurse practitioners should be able to provide good care for your child. If you have selected a health care provider prior to the birth of your child, you can simply continue to use him or her. It is most important that the health care provider be able to give you enough time to answer questions, and that he or she be knowledgeable in community resources. Your health care provider should also have an interest in monitoring your child's development and health, and must be willing to be a part of the team caring for her. It is vital for your health care provider to work closely with your baby's teachers, therapists, physician specialists, and family. Refer back to Chapter 3 for tips on dealing with health care providers.

Conclusion

Caring for a baby—any baby—is quite an imposing challenge. When that baby has Down syndrome and special needs, the task becomes more complicated. Though your baby is special, her daily care will be very much like that of other children. She can adjust to your life and fit in like other children. Information, patience, and persistence will help ease your new baby into a routine that is good for everyone. Use the books in the Reading List and seek the help of health care providers, teachers, and therapists. And always remember: your baby with Down syndrome, like every other baby, needs love, attention, and care.

Parent Statements

We feel it's very important to treat Julie normally. It's having normal expectations for behavior. For example, we put a lot of emphasis on eating properly, using her utensils properly, chewing properly, and things like that. We've had high expectations for her here at home, and her eating has been very good. Expecting normal behavior all the way around, even if you have to work harder at it, is the trick.

As far as little things go, I don't do too much differently with her except just pay more attention to her skin care. Other than that, I treat her like a normal baby; she didn't have any problems that I had to be careful about. As far as working with her goes, that was a major change because I was constantly striving to stimulate her. I was always playing and doing this and that, not only in our normal routine but making time to play with her, whereas before I probably would have done my housework or something. But that's been good too because I learned a lot about how to play with the baby.

The daily care of Josh has always been different from my other kids. It's been more intensive. It's carried a guilt element because we felt that there should be something else we should be doing all the time. We felt we should be making every moment a developmental laboratory.

Our baby has been nursed from when he was an infant so that's very lucky. He always nursed properly and started on solids at four months. He's twenty months now, and he feeds himself with a spoon. My husband is the best person to teach him how to eat because he really can give us the run-around if he wants to. We try not to let mealtimes become a battleground, but he likes testing. He's going through a testing phase, so we find him deliberately holding things over the side of his high chair and watching to see if we're going to say anything before he flings it over. But he can eat properly if he wants to.

When Laurie was two, she was a very plump little child. We put her on a diet, watched every speck she ate, and now she's fine. I think the Down syndrome makes her look heavier than she probably would otherwise. Her muscle tone has improved in the past few months, and she's getting good rotation in her trunk. So she'll be slim as can be in time. But her muscle mass is not good. I just really monitor her food. It's really hard when you have to switch gears after something like heart surgery. Before the surgery it was give, give, give, fortify, fortify—anything she wanted she got. A child gets in those behavior patterns easily.

We do have a hard time leaving her with a sitter. We just haven't felt comfortable doing that. I guess we just felt kind of protective. We didn't even go out for almost two years. Lately we have felt differently. We've left her with more people and she just gets along fine.

Toilet training Mike was no big deal. He took to it a little later than some other children, but he really had no more problems learning toileting than other kids, and in fact had fewer problems than some "normal" children of my friends.

Five

~~~~~~~~

Family Life With Your Baby

Marian H. Jarrett, Ed.D.*

You have undoubtedly thought about the changes in your life that the birth of your baby will bring. Many of these thoughts are happy ones, and rightfully so, because your baby will bring you great joy. But the arrival of a baby with Down syndrome also brings stress and strain on family members and on family relationships. Having a child with Down syndrome requires coping by the whole family. You will face the challenge of adjusting in your own way, but right from the start you should know that it can be done. Thousands of families can testify to that.

Today the future is bright for families of children with Down syndrome. So much has been learned to help families successfully raise their child. With early intervention for infants, special education programs, inclusion, better social acceptance, support groups, and vastly improved medical care, family life is dramatically better than it was even ten or twenty years ago. Families no longer need to struggle on their own.

Most parents worry about what having a child with Down syndrome will do to their families. One of the most common concerns is how well the child will fit into the family. Parents

---

*   Marian Jarrett holds a Doctorate in Education and is Assistant Professor of Teacher Preparation and Special Education, The George Washington University, Washington, D.C.

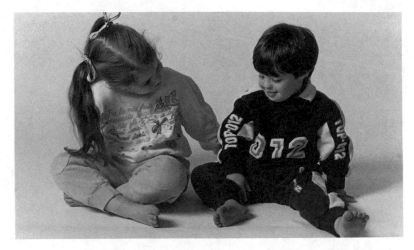

ask, "Will our child's behavior be so abnormal that everyday family life will be disrupted? Will I or my children be continually embarrassed by our child with Down syndrome? Will normal family fun come to an end?" These questions reflect the common concerns of new parents of babies with Down syndrome.

Parents also worry about how they can meet the challenge posed by a child with special needs. There is a great deal of work involved in raising any child with a disability, and raising a child with Down syndrome is no different. The challenge of fostering development, independence, and social ability is considerable, and parents naturally wonder how they can do all the work that is required. How can they give their special child all he needs and still meet their other responsibilities: to their other children, to their spouse, to their jobs, to themselves?

A major part of the worry that parents feel is fear of the unknown. But remember, other parents have faced the same fears and worries. They will tell you that raising a child with Down syndrome forced changes in their lives that involved hard work and considerable adjustment. They will also tell you that their child was a positive addition to the family and that they cannot imagine life without him or her.

Parents are the key to how well a family adjusts to having a family member with Down syndrome. Children, other family members, and friends follow the parents' cues. How you act toward your child sets the pattern for the whole family from the moment your baby is born.

Being the Parent of a Baby with Down Syndrome

Before the birth of your baby, you may have imagined child rearing would come naturally. But the parent of a baby with Down syndrome faces unique challenges, and what once seemed easy and natural now seems fraught with complications. You may ask yourself, "How can I feed this baby who struggles so much when he is being fed? Will I have to do special exercises to teach him to walk? Will he ever talk and will we understand what he says?" You may wonder how this baby can ever be a part of your family as worries about the future invade all your thoughts and activities.

All parents face worries and conflicting emotions in the early stages of their baby's life. Like parents of babies with Down syndrome, they worry about colic, feeding schedules, rashes, colds, and countless other details of child care. They soon learn to depend on love, acceptance, and discipline as the staples of good parenting. You will undoubtedly depend on these also in raising your child. Although this section focuses on those areas of family life that are *different* because your child is special, the goal for you is the same as for all families: integrating your child into your growing family as a valued, contributing member.

You may turn to your family and friends for help in meeting the challenge of bringing up your child. Also remember that your child's teacher and other professionals can be a tremendous source of support for you. The parent-professional partnership, which is discussed in Chapter 7, can be a great source of practical information on coping. Just having someone you can ask about problems or questions makes your daily work easier. Nagging uncertainties, worries, and questions can be dealt with quickly. More importantly, the advice of teachers and other professionals is based on the collective experience of many children and families. As a result, this advice can be very useful in offering you options for dealing with your own problems and worries.

Becoming Part of the Family

Right from the start, you should expect that your baby with Down syndrome will be a *part* of your family, not the center of it. Just because your child is special does not mean he should dominate family life. This is not good for your baby nor for the rest of the family. Your baby does have special needs and he will demand emotional and physical resources that other children might not demand. But remember, your goal is to balance all the competing demands so that everyone in the family can be an equal and contributing member. This is the same challenge that all parents face, whether they have a child with disabilities or not.

The relationship of each family member with the child with Down syndrome will be a reflection of your attitudes as parents. If you hold and cuddle and love your baby, if you voice your feelings of affection, if you face challenges in a positive manner, then other family members will too. As you begin the task of integrating your baby and his disability into your lives, you and all of your family will grow to love your baby more and more. That love will be your strongest ally, your strongest bond. Through patience and understanding your child can be a loved and loving member of your family.

In addition to a supportive environment, it is essential that your children have information. Leaving things unsaid will only send a confused and troubling message to your children. Tell them that their sibling has Down syndrome as soon as you think they are ready. Explain it on a level they can understand, and give them more information as they get older. Children have the ability to love their brother or sister unconditionally. You will be surprised at how much they understand and how easily they accept what most adults receive with shock and sadness.

If you accept your child with Down syndrome and are comfortable with him, he will fit into your family and your lifestyle. Your child will enjoy family mealtimes, outings, and going to school with other children. Your child may be able to receive most of his education in a school where he is included in a regular classroom with typically developing children. This can allow your child to learn from the example of the children in his regular classes. Working to make your child as much a part of the "normal" world in his

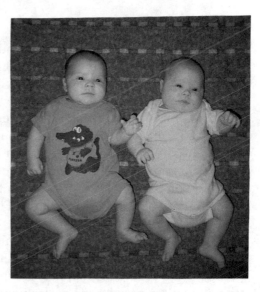

school and in your family life will help him tremendously. And the benefits of this are twofold. Not only will it help your child, but it will also help others in your child's world become more familiar and more comfortable with people with Down syndrome.

Take your child to the swimming pool, to the grocery store, to restaurants. Often the promise of "going out for spaghetti" can make a day go better, and the meal can be a special time for the entire family. Make sure your child participates in a variety of community activities, such as sports, Scouts, and art classes. Find things that he likes and can participate in with other children.

The medical problems that some babies with Down syndrome have can add to the stress a family experiences. Although the goal is to make your child an integral part of your family, medical needs may make this difficult. Parents sometimes need to focus their attention just on their child with Down syndrome. This is not unreasonable. It can happen in any family when a child is sick or has a special problem. Remember to let your other children be involved with their sibling. Encourage them to make hospital visits and to express their feelings. Above all, keep them informed. They will be concerned and will want to help.

Love and Acceptance

The birth of a baby with Down syndrome comes as a shock to most parents. In addition to the feelings of love and protection they have for their new baby, they also feel sadness and grief. These mixed feelings toward the baby often continue as the child grows. Do not hesitate to recognize these feelings within yourself and accept them without feeling guilty about them. No parent feels good about their child all the time.

Get to know your baby. Learn more about Down syndrome. Initially, you may be afraid to love your baby because you know so little about him and his condition. The closer you get to him, the more at ease you will become.

Today you can develop a relationship with your baby with confidence. Bolstered by the guidance and support of informed professionals, community support groups, and family and friends, you can provide an environment in which your child can grow to be a unique individual supported by your love.

Parents used to be told, "Just put him in an institution and forget about him." But children with Down syndrome have proven how well they respond to a stimulating and loving home. If you put a child in an institution, he will act like he belongs there; if you keep him at home and work with him, he will act like he belongs with you. Your relationship with your child— built on love and acceptance—is the key.

Some parents feel that they cannot keep their baby with Down syndrome at home. One alternative is to place the child for adoption. There are agencies with waiting lists of people who specifically want to adopt a baby with Down syndrome. Foster homes are also a viable alternative because children with Down syndrome benefit most from family life. The National Down Syndrome Congress has information about adoption.

Expectations

Babies with Down syndrome are born with a variety of physical and intellectual abilities. We know that these abilities are different from those of other children, but it is not possible to predict any child's full potential at an early age. At this point in your baby's life, do not set limits on what your child will or will not be able to do. Strive for that delicate balance between a realistic assessment of your child's development and the self-fulfilling prophecy of low achievement. Most of all, ensure that your child will lead a happy and useful life by providing appropriate support and training from an early age.

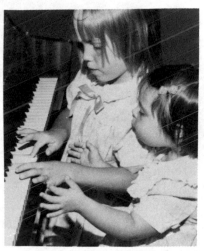

Parents spend more time with their young children than anyone else does, and their expectations can affect their children in tangible ways. For example, if you do not expect your child with Down syndrome to dress himself, he may not. Perhaps you unwittingly have not given him the chance. You may dress and undress him or simply help him too much because your expectations are too low.

Do not form your expectations in a vacuum and do not base them on stereotypes. Talk to doctors, teachers, therapists, and other parents of children with Down syndrome. It takes information and exposure to realistically set your expectations. More importantly, try not to look too far into the future. Focus on the next developmental skill; set short-term goals. After all, the future is made up of what your child learns along the way.

Limit Setting

Discipline is the parents' responsibility. Having a child with Down syndrome does not change that. You do not do your child a favor by failing to demand proper behavior because you feel sorry for him or because you think he cannot understand how to behave. If you allow your child to misbehave, you can be assured he will continue to misbehave. Your child's safety, social integration, and education depend on proper behavior. You owe it to your child to demand acceptable behavior.

Disciplining a child who has mental retardation may be a difficult thing for you to do. You may feel sorry for your child because he has Down syndrome. You may not be sure he understands what is expected of him. And, after giving him the same direction over and over, you may lose your patience and do it yourself. In public and with friends it is even harder. Not only do you not want to cause a scene, but you may not want to call attention to your child, to how difficult it appears to deal with him. However, the experience of many families is clear: discipline needs to be applied *consistently*. Children need to know what is, and what is not, acceptable conduct in *all* situations. Firmness and consistency work best; don't take the easy way out for reasons of convenience, embarrassment, or frustration. Unless you can teach your child safe and acceptable behavior, he may always be dependent on you.

The social development of children and adults with Down syndrome is often more advanced than their level of mental development. Give your child every chance to succeed in life by teaching him to behave the way you expect his brothers and sisters to behave. Set limits and be consistent in enforcing them. And remember, emphasize the positive. Praise and affection are the most powerful motivators for good behavior.

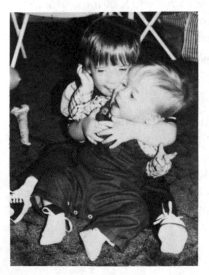

If your child can make the connection between his behavior and the consequences you might impose, removing him from the scene, placing him in a "time out" chair for a few minutes, or denying him a later pleasure are good tactics to try. Be sure that you clearly state your expectations for his behavior. "No hitting. Tell Ben 'My turn'" lets your child know what not to do and gives him an acceptable alternative.

Once he understands, you can explain briefly and unemotionally that if he misbehaves, then something will happen.

An extremely effective method of discipline is positive reward. For a young child, a big hug and "I like the way you play!" can go a long way in achieving acceptable behavior. For older children, you might try a reward chart with a star for each time he plays in the yard without throwing the ball over the fence or takes a bath without soaking the bathroom. Distraction can be effective also. If you child is doing something inappropriate, you might try suggesting something else you know will interest him.

For some children, the positive approach is the only one that consistently gets results. Your child may not understand why he is being punished. He may "dig in his heels" when you get angry. You may find that he responds better when you change your expression to a pleasant one, make your voice encouraging, and explain with excitement what he needs to do. This can move him in the direction you want to go without a prolonged battle which you might win, but leaves both you and your child in no mood to enjoy an activity.

An important consideration in disciplining your child is how others will handle him. With babysitters, grandparents, relatives, and friends, there is often the opportunity for your discipline to be undermined. It will be necessary for you to politely yet firmly let others know that discipline is important to you and to your child. Explain to them what conduct is acceptable and what is not. Help them understand and enlist their help. Firmness and consistency are not always easy to maintain, but they will pay off.

When setting expectations for your child's behavior, you must learn to give him enough time to process information. Do not expect instant responses or fast transitions from one activity to another. It is possible that he needs a little extra time to understand your wishes and to decide on his own response. What may appear to be resistance or stubbornness may simply be an inability to cope with your verbal demands or to deal with a transition. Some children find a change in routine a difficult emotional step and feel anxiety in moving from one activity to another. What you encounter may result less from "I don't want

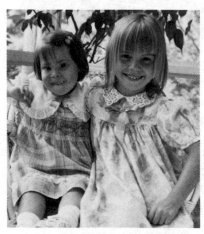

to do it" stubbornness and more from your child enjoying what he is doing and feeling anxious about being asked to do something else. If you are faced with a pattern of resistance, you can often break through it by offering a more interesting and exciting alternative. For example, suggest your child kick a ball into an overturned garbage can instead of toward the street or wonder aloud if all his bath toys will fit in the tub at once. You may have to observe your child and consider his developmental level and his ability to understand in order to distinguish between his resistance to reasonable expectations and his inability to process your demands. You as his parent will be in the best position to judge.

Independence

It is natural to feel that your child is particularly vulnerable because he has Down syndrome. It is a natural reaction to feel sorry for your child and to want to protect him. But for the sake of his future you must treat him as normally as possible. Your child needs to learn independence and responsibility. He needs to feel good about himself and what he can do.

Your job begins early in teaching your child self-help skills such as dressing and feeding himself. Give your child the opportunity to do things for himself. Don't rush to help him before you give him the chance to try something on his own. Encourage and praise him along the way and reward him with a big hug for a job well done.

Your child will likely be involved in an education or therapy program at an early age and will need to be "on his own" in many of these situations. Don't let your child's crying tempt you to give up on a new school or program that may be strange to him. Give him time to adjust. Children usually adjust well and enjoy school.

Expose your child to new situations whenever possible. Provide him with a variety of experiences and help him adjust to what is new and different. Take him to the zoo, introduce him to a sandbox, let him explore the local shopping mall. Give him responsibilities and chores within the family. When he is a preschooler, insist that he pick up his toys, but help him put them in the toy box or on the shelf. As he gets older, build on the things he enjoys. Maybe he can dust the furniture, take out the newspapers for recycling, help you work in the yard. Take the time to teach him and make sure that he can be successful at whatever task you ask him to do. When all the family works together, include your child with Down syndrome. Like all of us, he needs to feel like a valued member of the family. Think positively about what your child can do. Feel positive about his capabilities. Increase your child's self-esteem by giving him the opportunity to succeed within the secure confines of the family. This will help prepare him to move out into the larger world of friends, school, work, and community.

If your baby has a congenital heart defect, you may not be able to treat him as you would any other baby. Frequent trips to the hospital for cardiac studies, the risk of respiratory infection, and difficulty in feeding will necessitate extra care and caution on your part. Provide this care and protect your baby wisely, but be ready to allow him to move out into the world as soon as he is able. To be sure, this is not easy. Conflicting emotions and real medical concerns intensify the natural urge to protect your child and complicate the necessary process of letting go.

Brothers and Sisters of Children with Down Syndrome

Being the brother or sister of a child with Down syndrome is special. In many subtle and not-so-subtle ways your other children's lives will be different now that they have a special sibling. But do not assume that this difference is all bad. Far from it. Having a sibling with Down syndrome is stressful and enriching, frustrating and fun, worrisome and rewarding. Most of all, it is very much like being the sibling of any other child, complete with all the annoyances and joys. This section reviews the effects—both good and bad—that children with Down syndrome have on their siblings, and focuses on what you, the parent, can do to help all your children build healthy relationships with one another.

Children's Feelings

From the time they are old enough to understand, your other children will have thoughts and feelings about their special sibling. At first, they may perceive only that it takes their brother or sister longer to do things like walk or talk. Later, they will begin to understand that their brother or sister has a disability. What follows is a summary of the thoughts and feelings typically experienced by siblings of children with Down syndrome.

Pre-School. Children are very perceptive, so it is possible for your other children to react to the anxiety you feel about your baby with Down syndrome. At this age they are unlikely to recognize any difference in their special sibling or understand what Down syndrome is, but pre-schoolers may perceive developmental differences and try in their own way to help teach skills. They want to help. Mostly this is an age when children fall in love with their sibling and want to help take care of him.

Ages Four to Six. As children become more sophisticated they often begin to wonder what is "wrong" with their sibling. They may worry about catching Down syndrome or worry that something is different about them as well. Additionally, they often feel guilty about any negative thoughts they may have toward their special sibling. For example, anger caused by frustration—a perfectly normal response for young children at times—can cause feelings of guilt. Sometimes children try to compensate for their special sibling's problems by trying to be especially exemplary themselves. They become excessively helpful and obedient beyond limits that are good for them, for your family, or for your child with Down syndrome.

Ages Six to Twelve. Children at these ages often have conflicting emotions. On the one hand, they can feel good about being needed by their special sibling, and on the other hand, can consider their sibling a nuisance. They may respond to teasing of their sibling by becoming hostile toward the culprit or by being protective. At the same time they may be resentful of any extra work imposed on them as a result of their sibling's special needs. Your preoccupation with your child with Down syndrome can be viewed by other children as "babying," which they may consider unfair.

Ages Twelve to Sixteen. During this important period of adolescent development, your child's social life often causes some very normal problems. Teenagers can feel embarrassed by their families. When friends and dates come to your house, your teenager may feel quite embarrassed by your child with Down syndrome. Your teenager will love his or her sibling and care about him, but just as certainly will want to exercise freedom and independence. This is a time when responsibilities imposed on your other children—including responsibility for your child with Down syndrome—may be resented. Concerns over the future also can arise. Your other children may worry whether they will have to take responsibility for their special sibling in later years and whether their own children will have Down syndrome.

These are just some of the possible feelings your child with Down syndrome may trigger in your other children. Emotions come in every shape and size, and each child's feelings are unique. But some feelings seem universal. Love, fear, jealousy, resentment, anger, pride, and frustration are present at some time in children, as they are in adults. The central challenge for a caring parent is to deal with these many genuine—and conflicting—human emotions.

Dealing with Your Children's Emotions

Just as you experience stress as the parent of a child with Down syndrome, your other children will also find it stressful to be the sibling of a child with disabilities. But the strongest fac-

tor in their adjustment will be *your* reaction. They will follow
your lead in interacting with their brother or sister. Keep in
mind, however, that, like you, they will have conflicting emotions about their sibling. It would be easier if children clearly
showed their feelings, but often children do not, or cannot, express how they are feeling about life with their sibling. Parents
must be emotional detectives, deciphering their children's emotions from clues in their behavior. First and foremost, dealing effectively with emotions requires observation and listening.

Information. Children can deal better with their sibling
with Down syndrome if they have information. You should be
the main source of this information. Even if they do not ask,
give them information. As with other subjects, give them information appropriate to their age level and expand it as they grow.
There are many fine books written specifically for siblings of
children with Down syndrome and other disabilities. The Reading List at the back of this book includes some of these books.

Even with an explanation of what Down syndrome is and
what it means to have mental retardation, your children may
still be concerned and worried. They may worry about catching
Down syndrome, about having children of their own, and about
caring for their sibling in the future. Continue to provide information and to reassure your children. Their sibling does not
have to be a burden. Be ready to debunk the myths they may
hear by giving them the facts.

Communication. It is important that you encourage and
even prod your children to talk about the feelings they have for
their sibling. Let them know it is normal to feel as they do and
that it is healthy to express themselves. If possible, let them
join with other siblings of children with disabilities to work
through their feelings. Sibling groups are sponsored by a variety
of organizations, and are listed in this book's Resource Guide.
Urge your children to take advantage of the opportunity to sort
out what they are feeling and experiencing.

Children get angry, annoyed, frustrated—as we all do. Sometimes they fight. But when a sibling with Down syndrome is the
cause of that anger, young children can experience great difficulty. Sometimes out of sympathy for their parents or their sib-

ling, children feel guilty about their anger. They may begin to resent their sibling or avoid interacting with him. They may withdraw, not only from their sibling, but from other family members also. As a parent, it is vital for you to let your children know that it is sometimes reasonable to get angry with their sibling and to vent that anger. All of your children need to communicate their anger over things like broken toys or misplaced keepsakes. Protecting your child with Down syndrome from the often well-deserved wrath of his siblings cuts off communication and forces feelings underground. Anger is a natural part of family life. Every member is a target from time to time. Having a child with Down syndrome should not change that.

Balance. It is important that you balance the needs of all of your children. Encourage all of them to succeed and to fulfill themselves. Do not give all of your attention to your child with Down syndrome. It is not healthy for one child to dominate parental attention in family life. Instead, you need to skillfully juggle the many demands on your time and attention.

Do not allow your special child to become overly dependent on his siblings. Rather, encourage your children to take an active part in their sibling's educational and therapeutic programs. They, too, will become emotionally attached to their brother and will rejoice in each independent step he takes. And, remember to allow them to do this *as a brother or sister*. Do not press them into the role of parent, even if they seem willing to assume it. Do not expect that an older child will feed, bathe, and dress his brother every day. Do not insist that his brother always go along to the grocery store or the drugstore when you send your teenager on an errand. And do not insist that your child change his plans in order to babysit his brother. This can breed long-standing resentment. Better to sit down with all family members and work out how you will share responsibilities for your child with Down syndrome so that each person's needs are met.

Organization. With all that is urged upon parents of babies with Down syndrome—early intervention, monitoring for medical problems, all the normal baby-care responsibilities—it is easy to unintentionally overlook your other children's needs.

There is only so much of you and only so many hours in a day. Try to organize your time. With a child with special needs, the challenge is a little greater, but it can be done.

Children do not conveniently schedule their crises. They get hurt, upset, or excited on their own time, and when they do, they demand your immediate and full attention. Parents often cannot control their own schedules, but there are a few things you can do to keep things running reasonably smoothly. Here is a short list of ideas:

- Keep track of the amount of time spent with each child. Try to spend some individual time with each child and your spouse. And leave some time for yourself.
- Whenever possible, schedule the time that must be spent exclusively with your child with Down syndrome at times when your other children are not at home or are otherwise occupied.
- When your children are at home, organize group play that includes all your children. Let your older children lead and your younger children follow.
- Keep your children busy. Schedule play times, visits to friends' houses, and outings to the park. But avoid over-doing it—avoid the syndrome of rushing around all the time, trying to cram too much into each day.
- Don't try to do it all yourself. Organize car pools and play groups. Pay a babysitter or trade with another parent.

Individuality. Just as this book encourages you to treat your child with Down syndrome as an individual, it is equally important to do the same for your other children. They need lives outside their family. They need to experience peer friendship, social acceptance, and nonfamily responsibilities. Their identity cannot be limited just to being the sibling of a brother or sister with Down syndrome. Provide them with activities away from home, with their own friends. Encourage them to pursue their own interests and talents and to exercise their independence. Build their self-esteem just as you would with your child with Down syndrome. Children with balanced lives will be far better adjusted to their family, as well as more supportive of both you and their sibling.

Your expectations of your children can make a difference. Expect, demand, and work to build and maintain normal family relationships. Allow your other children to act like children. And let them know that you expect your child with Down syndrome to behave appropriately. Siblings resent favored treatment accorded to others. It is important to both your other children and your child with Down syndrome that you require him to help take care of himself and to contribute in helping with the family chores. Don't settle for less.

Specialness. In addition to encouraging your other children to lead their own lives, it is also very important to give them a sense of their own specialness. Let them know that because their sibling is special, so are they—in a very positive way. Most siblings naturally feel good about being needed by their special sibling. As parents you can reinforce those feelings. Praise their compassion, the extra work they do around the house, and the extra coping required of them. Make them feel that their efforts are recognized and appreciated.

Dealing with Problems

Although society has become far more sensitive and compassionate toward people with disabilities, there is no guarantee that your children will not occasionally be wounded by teasing or cruel remarks. Siblings of children with Down syndrome know their brother or sister is different, and they often are quite protective. When feelings are hurt, parents usually get the job of soothing. Good family communication is a must in these situations.

When adults say insensitive things, siblings of special children can have surprising responses. They may think the adult is ignorant or mean. But if the adult is someone they know and trust, confusion and uncertainty can arise. Parents need to confront these incidents head-on, with facts. Reassure and support your children with information and understanding.

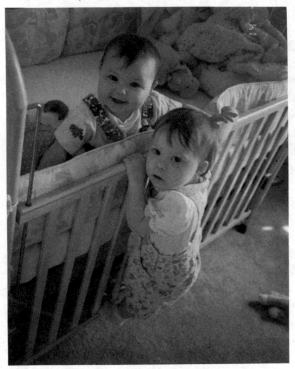

Dealing with the cruel remarks and teasing of children can be more difficult than dealing with those of adults. As children grow, peer acceptance and social interaction increase in importance. Special kids can sometimes embarrass their siblings, who in turn may alienate their own friends in defense of their special sibling. In addition to encouraging them to express their feelings and offering them reassurance, parents should make sure that their other children have time to be on their own, with their own friends.

Children sometimes repeat the comments and teasing they hear and see at school. When parents overhear teasing or get a report from their children, they sometimes get angry and want to set things right. Children, however, need to learn to cope with life on their own. Fight the urge to rescue. Children can develop their own effective ways of coping and they can do it without losing their love for their special sibling or the friendship of their peers. Talk to your children. Urge them to talk about how they felt when they were teased. Talk with them about reasons why someone might make such comments. Help them think of ways they might respond and choose how they will react in the future. Help them to think of ways to talk about their sibling to help explain his differences to their friends and playmates. Often a simple explanation that it is harder for him to talk or that it takes him longer to learn something is all it takes. Your children will have to deal with others' reactions to their sibling for a long time, so avoid fighting their battles for them. All of you will feel better when they find the way that is comfortable for them.

Counseling can help children who experience trouble in coping with their sibling. Talking to someone outside the family, such as an objective, caring professional, can help a great deal. Not all problems need to be solved within the family. Sometimes giving your child room to adjust with the help of a counselor can accomplish what you cannot. Do not be too afraid—or too proud—to seek help. Pediatricians, therapists, special educators, and school counselors are frequently asked by parents for names of counselors who are especially good in working with children. Also remember that you have the experience of other parents and of the organizations listed in this book to guide you in finding someone who can help.

The Future

As your other children grow and mature they will begin to think about their future with their special sibling. Questions about responsibility and care will be asked. Again, you need to provide facts. Let your children know that they will not need to be responsible for their adult sibling with Down syndrome unless they choose to be. With the increased social integration of people with Down syndrome, there are a wide variety of community residential and employment programs available so that siblings need not fear life-long burdens.

Your children and their future will likely be affected by their sibling with Down syndrome. Being the sibling of a child with Down syndrome can cause problems and frustrations, but at the same time it can warm the hearts of your children for a lifetime. Remember that having a sibling with disabilities has its good points. Many siblings develop a strong capacity for love and acceptance of someone who is different. They may develop a sense not only of social understanding, but also of social responsibility. They may choose a career in one of the helping professions in an effort to make things better for those who are different. Your children may also develop a sense of specialness about your family and the special ties that bind you together.

This section has emphasized the importance of communication between parents and their children. Remember, parents are not infallible and do not always have all the answers: they hurt, they worry, they feel frustrated. It is not always necessary to put up a cheerful front for the sake of your kids. Let your children know that you do not have all the answers, that you need *their* support, that you are all in this together. Children usually surprise parents with how much they understand and how much they care. Let your children share in the effort of coping with a child with Down syndrome.

Your Child with Down Syndrome and Your Marriage

The greatest source of support you have as parents of a child with Down syndrome is each other. Although your child is a source of stress and strain for each of you and for your relationship, you can help one another in dealing with this unexpected event in your lives. The starting place is to identify ways in which you have coped with other difficult situations in your lives. Use these same strategies in dealing with the needs of your child with Down syndrome.

If your relationship with your spouse is strong, your marriage can probably withstand the additional stress imposed on it by the birth of your child. In fact, some parents feel that their baby has drawn them closer together. They speak of their awareness of their parental roles and of their responsibility to their child: "We feel we must stick together and support each other in each new crisis related to him."

One of the best ways to support one another is to openly share your feelings about your child with Down syndrome. Remember that you will feel love, hate, anger, fear, guilt—a full spectrum of conflicting emotions. It is perfectly normal to have these feelings, and you should let your spouse know that it is okay for him or her to have them too. If you share and acknowledge these feelings, you can work through them together, or together you can seek the help of others to aid you in this important process. You may find it helpful to talk to a friend, another parent, a priest, rabbi, or minister, a psychologist, or a counselor.

When your baby is young, he may be like any other baby in terms of the amount of care and attention needed. But as a toddler, his physical and educational needs will increasingly infringe on the time and energy you can devote to one another. One parent of an infant with Down syndrome spoke about the influence of the infant on his relationship with his wife:

> *The most difficult thing has been finding the time to be alone together, to work on our relationship. This is true of all parents with infants, but especially with special-needs infants because we have so many extra doctor appointments. Also, we must work much harder to stimulate our infant. We really don't spend more time playing with her, but more energy. It takes more psychological energy to get her to respond.*

Like all parents, you worry about your child's future. You think about his education, his ability to participate in sports and other peer activities, his prospects for employment, and his ability to live independently. Although you will want to find more information about each of these subjects at the appropriate time, you must also learn to live one day at a time. Learn to focus on small steps in your child's development. He now rolls to get what he wants, he stays dry all night, he sits through a whole story at circle time, he plays soccer with the kids at recess. Learn to enjoy today with your child. Celebrate life's small triumphs.

Earlier in this chapter the statement was made that your special child should not be the center of your family. If you allow that to happen, anger and resentment can build up in you and in other family members. Likewise, your child should not be the center of one parent or partner's life or the sole responsibility of one parent or partner. Each of you should share in the care, stimulation, education, and the pleasure of loving your

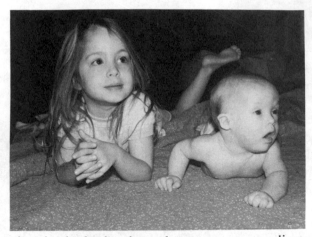

child. You need to decide what arrangement works best for you. Even though Mom or Dad is tired at the end of the day, a short play session with his child or a fun time in the bath tub can be a great stress reliever. When your child is unable to enjoy activities that his siblings like, Mom may want to go off to the museum with the other children while Dad stays home and takes him to the grocery store.

Your child will require extra time and attention and you may feel you need to be a "super" parent. You and your spouse may have radically different expectations or may not be able to support one another in dealing with your child's special needs. Perhaps your feelings of anger or guilt will cause you to do everything for your child to make his life easier. This will likely leave you exhausted and frustrated—and not available to your other children or to your spouse or partner. Don't try to do it all. It's okay to let things slip once in awhile. Take time for yourself. Take a good look at what you are doing and why. Talk to your spouse; nothing replaces open, honest communication. Get help if you need it. Talk to your minister or a family counselor. Read books about parenting and relationships and find ways to strengthen your marriage and your family.

Conclusion

It isn't easy having a child with Down syndrome in the family. In many ways it is richly rewarding, but it is also stressful—on children, on parents, and on the whole family. There is no formula for coping perfectly with Down syndrome. Love, communication, acceptance, and the steadfast belief that your family will in the end thrive are your best bets to ensure a healthy and rewarding family life.

There are many books on families that have children with special needs. As you begin the task of integrating your child with Down syndrome into your family, reading about the experiences of others can help you a great deal. So can talking to other parents of children with Down syndrome. Their advice, based on what has worked best for them, can be very helpful. Just sharing similar problems and triumphs can help put your life in perspective. Most importantly, remember that you, your spouse, and your whole family are all in this together. Before long, your child with Down syndrome will just be part of the team.

Parent Statements

My relatives were all very good. They were amazing, actually. All my brothers and my sister just concentrated on him; they just responded to him completely. And my mother acted as if there was nothing different about him at all.

～〜〜〜〜〜〜〜

Our relatives' reactions have varied. One relative was a little bit condescending about it. He said, "Oh, he's one of God's children; it's okay." He was trying to comfort us, but I think he took the wrong approach.

～〜〜〜〜〜〜〜

Christopher has made us a family. He's a little child and you know, it doesn't really matter that he has Down syndrome. Mothers and fathers and children make families and he's been in every way affectionate and childlike and all the things that children are. That's what makes a family.

～〜〜〜〜〜〜〜

We decided that any child would have to fit into our lives. For example, Laurie has so many appointments and needs, but I had originally decided to go back to work. I adjusted it and went back part time. I decided I needed that for myself. We still had to go out at night. We still had to have time alone.

I think every child with Down syndrome should have a person who energizes him, and I don't think it should be a parent. A sibling, an aunt, a next-door neighbor. I've now met three kids who have a person like that and all three kids seem to have a spirit to them.

Our family has been somewhat varied in their reaction. I think there was a lot of sorrow. But I think our own attitude helped a lot of the family work it out. Our attitude of "We're just crazy about this baby" helped everyone a lot.

We treat him generally just like another kid. If we want to go out shopping, okay, he's going to go shopping. He eats what we eat. We don't try to shield him. He has to live in the world. The world's not going to change to accommodate him. The more he is out in the world, the more he will be able to adjust to it.

We had a very interesting experience about three weeks ago. An old friend has a son who is five. We went to visit them for the first time in about two years. They decided not to say anything to their son about Josh having Down syndrome, and to just see what happened. Their son treated him just like a regular kid; it didn't bother him that Josh didn't talk much. They got along great. Maybe if you don't prejudice them, kids accept each other as they are.

We have two kids, and one of them has extremely high intelligence, and the other has Down syndrome. It's tough to switch gears sometimes. It takes a lot of patience, and I don't think I have as much as I'd like to have.

I didn't really feel a sense of mourning or disappointment until recently. It all evolved around placement in schools and integration into the neighborhood. I realized that I was working so much harder to make things easier for this child than with the other two children. It was a mourning; she wasn't a regular kid and I sometimes find myself wishing that it were a little easier.

We like to keep strict tabs on her behavior. We find ourselves saying, "That's cute at four but it's not going to be so cute at eight."

We use discipline with a lot of consistency, a lot of patience, and never expecting more than she's able to comprehend at the moment.

Sometimes I worry about him because he gets so much attention from adults. He has teachers coming to the house and fawning on him an hour at a time. And he's charming his way through school. He's got the director of the school he goes to just eating out of the palm of his hand. I'm afraid he'll get away with things just by being cute.

We've tried different things for discipline. First, we tried the punitive way for misbehavior. We had a relative who was in special ed who said, "Oh you must try behavior modification and every time he throws his food you have to keep him from it for five minutes." And so we ended up with him getting very bad tempered and starving and everybody unable to eat their meal because they were too upset by his screaming. It didn't achieve a single thing. We discussed the problem with his educator and decided to try modeling what he should do. It worked instantly. We picked up all the food he threw down and put it in his hand and told him to put it back on the table. He did it and he was so pleased with himself that he started doing it normally.

I'm kind of a strong disciplinarian and I try to keep the same standards of discipline for all three kids. But with Julie you can't let too much time elapse between the event and saying, "No, this is something we don't do."

It's important for Laurie's sister to always be able to express her feelings, and she shouldn't just have to mirror our feelings. Her feelings are going to be different, and we shouldn't feed her our feelings so that those are the only acceptable ones.

When we found out we were going to have twins—a boy and a girl—we thought we were going to have the perfect little family. Then when it turned out that our daughter had Down syndrome, it seemed like Fate was laughing in our face for even daring to think that we were going to live happily ever after. We were crushed. After a while, though, we began to see the positive side of things. They could still be great playmates and friends, we realized, and our son could be a terrific model for our daughter to imitate. We would always know exactly where she stood developmentally by comparing her skills to his.

There's a lot of sibling rivalry that would be there anyway, I think. But we had the teacher come in every week, and the older one slowly caught on that there was something unusual about his brother. He may have become resentful over the amount of attention his brother got.

Our oldest daughter is a real companion to Julie. But the middle one feels just caught next to this little kid who's a pain in the neck sometimes. But a four-year-old sibling would be a pain in the neck even if she didn't have Down syndrome.

Josh's older brother hasn't seemed to have had problems with teasing from other kids. His friends come here all the time. He's got three or four guys who seem to be here every evening. They take Josh as one of the givens of the house.

I was a little worried about how Hope would react when we brought our new baby home from the hospital, dethroning her from her only-child status. For the most part, though, Hope is as gentle and sweet with the baby as any toddler could be. She gives the baby lots of kisses, shakes rattles for her, tries to feed her a bottle, "shh's" people when the baby is sleeping.

The thing that has taken us most by surprise is integrating into the neighborhood. We have very nice neighbors and they think the world of Julie, but they have their own four-year-old children who are normal, competent, capable children who play together real well. There's nothing malicious, you just see the childhood neighborhood going by without her. Unlike fighting to get your kid in the school system, where you become an advocate, you can't do that with the neighborhood. You can't tell the neighbor kids to play with your kid.

◦◦◦◦◦◦◦◦◦

Will is not a very good playmate, and that is a big problem. Even with inclusion, he has not developed real friendships. I wish there were more children with disabilities in the school system. All the benefits of inclusion would not take away from his being able to become friends with other children who might share his interests, even if they are only watching a video together.

◦◦◦◦◦◦◦◦◦

I think if you had a weak marriage, Down syndrome would come as an obstacle between you. There were times when it was hard for my husband. Until she was about two, I was really involved in meeting all her needs. It took time away from him.

◦◦◦◦◦◦◦◦◦

There are positives and negatives as to the effects on our marriage and family, and on balance it comes out positive. It's more of a workload. It's the struggle with education, a whole new dimension of work that has to be split up. On the other hand, it brought a whole new quality dimension to our life. We both wind up feeling that our family is so much richer. I sometimes think life would be boring if we had all normal kids. Normal seems so boring.

◦◦◦◦◦◦◦◦◦

One of the things about marriage is that when you have kids, you assume that those kids are going to be a part of your life for eighteen to twenty years and then you're going to go back to being a couple. But when your kid has Down syndrome, it dawns on you that this kid could be around forever. Then you go through a stage of realizing that that isn't the case—that a kid with mental retardation can grow up and have a life too. Then it's a different emotion, like we don't want her to leave. I know that separation is coming, but it's going to be tough.

～～～～～～～～～

Having a baby with Down syndrome didn't diminish the desire to have more children. But the thing was, I had a hysterectomy as a result of her birth. We decided immediately to adopt more children. We definitely would hate the idea of our daughter not having any other siblings. So we have planned an adoption. The baby will come from Honduras and everyone keeps saying "How do you know it won't have something wrong with it?" And so we say, "Well, we could have produced one ourselves that had something wrong with it."

～～～～～～～～～

I can only deal with one day at a time. I have a real hard time planning too far ahead. I don't mean that I muddle through each day, but I can only plan one day in advance. I think someday I'll evolve out of that and everything will be better and I can plan ahead like I used to.

Six

∿∿∿∿∿∿

Your Baby's Development

French McConnaughey, M.Ed.* and
Patricia O. Quinn. M.D.**

One of life's great pleasures is watching your children grow
and learn. Sharing in their first steps and first words makes the
hard work of being a parent all worthwhile. As babies progress
from total dependence to walking out the front door ready for
school, parents feel great pride. All of this miraculous change,
wonderful growth, and learning is commonly called "development."

Every child learns and grows. So will your baby with Down
syndrome. Like every other baby, she can provide you with
great joy as you watch her growth and development. She will
need your help, and she may develop more slowly, but she will
learn, change, and grow. You will be excited and proud.

This chapter introduces the important subject of "development." It provides you with an overview along with an introduction to some of the specific developmental needs babies with
Down syndrome have. As parents, it is important for you to have

---

* French McConnaughey holds a Masters in Special Education. She is
currently the Director of the Concord Hill School in Chevy Chase,
Maryland.

** Patricia O. Quinn, M.D., is a developmental pediatrician in the
Washington, D.C. area. She is the author of *Putting on the Brakes: Young
People's Guide to Understanding Attention Deficit Disorder*, *"Putting on the Brakes
Activity Book for Young People with ADHD*, and *ADD and the College Student: A
Guide for High School* and *College Students with ADD*.

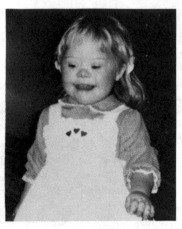

a basic understanding of development and to appreciate the important role you can play in enabling your child to maximize her potential.

Parents who get involved in their baby's development truly share in their child's first steps and first words. Studies show that babies whose parents are actively involved in their development make better progress than babies whose parents are not. There is no substitute for direct parental involvement, and with the help of teachers and other professionals, parents can make a tremendous difference. The challenges are great, and there is much hard work involved, but the rewards—pride and joy in your child's accomplishments—are just as great.

What Is "Development?"

Human development is the complex process of growing and acquiring skills. The foundations of development are in a baby's genetic make-up and her environment. Development is a lifelong process that is a result of the complex interplay of biological, psychological, cultural, and environmental factors. With each person influenced by so many variables, it is logical that everyone develops in a unique way.

The endpoint of development is not a predetermined and unchanging level of ability. Instead, development is an evolving process, subject to both positive and negative influences. If we view development as a process by which an individual realizes her potential, then we are presented with the challenge of how we can best foster that process.

Development can and should be monitored in order to optimize positive factors, such as personality traits and a supportive family environment, and to reduce the impact of negative influences, such as heart conditions, health problems, and other chronic illnesses. Although the developmental process cannot be totally controlled, it can be dramatically affected by direct intervention.

The development of a baby with Down syndrome will be affected by her extra chromosome. Her genetic make-up establishes a preliminary blueprint for development; it does not predetermine the end result. Genes have created the disabilities seen in Down syndrome; growth and learning in concert with positive psychological, cultural, and environmental factors can help lessen the impact of those disabilities.

What is "Normal" Development?

Development occurs in a sequence that is miraculously organized. As your child achieves each new skill, or *developmental milestone*, she lays the foundation for the next step, as increasingly sophisticated skills are acquired. For example, those cute "coos" and babbles are the precursors of words, which eventually become sentences.

Because each baby's development is the result of many factors, there is a broad range that is viewed as "normal" development. For example, one child may learn to walk three months earlier than another, but say her first words three months later than her peers. One child may move step by step through the sitting-crawling-walking sequence while another skips crawling altogether. Each child has her own learning profile that crisscrosses the "normal developmental scale." For parents it is helpful to use developmental milestones and sequences as a guide to chart the long-range course. These milestones, however, are not the only recipe for development. As you watch your child learn and grow you will begin to appreciate her individual learning style, strengths, and weaknesses. With that knowledge you will be better equipped to anticipate where help may be needed to facilitate development.

The Six Areas of Development

The process of development has been described in many different ways. One common approach is to divide the process into six areas: 1) gross motor, 2) fine motor, 3) language, 4) cognition, 5) social, and 6) self-help. Although each area has its own developmental sequence, they all are closely interrelated. Progress in one area affects progress in others in obvious and subtle ways. For example, your child's ability to speak will be a major factor in her social and play skills; her finger dexterity will affect her self-help skills significantly.

While it is useful to look at development by breaking it down into categories, remember that children should be viewed as a whole. All areas of development are interrelated. Fine motor abilities build on gross motor skills. Self-help skills are dependent on motor development. Social and self-help skills often take place only after both motor and cognitive foundations have been laid. As you can see, growth in one area dramatically influences growth in others. Avoid preoccupation with any single area and strive for overall balance.

Gross Motor. Through gross motor development, a baby learns to move her body by using her large muscles, including those in the legs, arms, and abdomen. Sitting up, crawling, walking, and climbing are all important gross motor skills. These skills allow your baby to move around, explore her world, and lay a foundation for growth in other areas.

Fine Motor. Development in this area involves the skills your baby learns in order to control her small and detailed movements. Typical fine motor muscles include the muscles in the fingers and hands. Skills like picking up a small object, using the index finger to poke and probe, and squeezing soft objects are all important fine motor skills. The control of eye muscles as well as facial and tongue movements are also important parts of the fine motor repertoire.

Language. Learning to communicate is one of the most important and remarkable accomplishments of childhood. Language development is usually divided into two areas: *receptive language* and *expressive language*. Receptive language is the ability to understand words and gestures. Expressive language is the

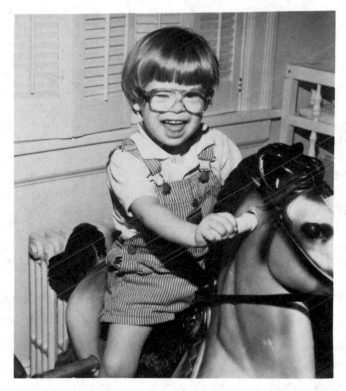

ability to use gestures, words, and written symbols to communicate. In the acquisition of language skills, the understanding of a word—a receptive skill—usually precedes the ability to express that word. It is not uncommon to hear a parent say "my baby understands more than she says." In analyzing your own language you will realize that you have a far greater receptive vocabulary than the number of words you use in everyday conversation. That is true for all children.

Cognition. Cognition has been the subject of many books, and its definition the object of much debate. In a practical study of development, cognition can be viewed as the ability to reason and solve problems. In babies these skills include the ability to understand object permanence (that objects do not cease to exist when they are out of sight), to understand cause and effect, and to draw conclusions from direct experience and later from observation or recall. These complex and abstract concepts take time to learn, and babies usually learn them from play. Finding hidden objects teaches object permanence; spilling a container teaches cause and effect; stacking blocks provides the opportunity to experience the concepts of size and shape. Each of these skills helps build the important foundation of concepts your child needs to understand how the world works, how objects relate to one another, and how she can manipulate her environment.

Social. Social development is the ability to function in relationship to others. From birth onward, babies learn how to respond appropriately to themselves and relate to others. They learn how to play with people and objects, become attached to people, and learn ways to assert their individual independence. As toddlers, they begin to function in a society of peers. These are the foundation skills that enable babies to mature into functioning members of society.

Self-Help. Self-help is the ability to take care of oneself, and is an important area of development. At birth, babies are totally dependent on others for their care. As they grow and develop, they acquire skills like feeding, dressing, and toileting which allow them to be more independent.

A seventh area—*sensory processing*—is very important to a child's overall development. It is not, however, usually considered a separate area of development. Sensory processing acts as an umbrella covering all areas and is defined as the ability of a child to process sensations like touch, sound, light, smell, and movement. These skills are refined as babies grow, and they affect all other areas of development. In the beginning, the sensory system functions primarily to protect your baby by reflexes like gagging; eventually it becomes more sophisticated and can perform other functions like discriminating between textures and tastes of foods. And a well functioning sensory system is necessary for good development. For example, the development of cognitive skills depends on your child's ability to see and hear.

The Sequence of Development

Asking questions about development is natural for all parents. "What will my baby do and when should she do it? How can I help my baby learn the skills she needs?" By learning the basic sequence of human development—the progression of learning skills—you can begin to put your child's growth into perspective and play a critical role in aiding her growth and learning.

The First Three Years

The changes that occur during the first three years of life are extraordinary. Your newborn is completely dependent on you and must rely on you for survival. Initially, her behavior is most often the result of reflexes and sensations over which she has little control. By the time of her third birthday, she has developed general control over her body and has become a social being. She can survive somewhat independently, solve problems, and use the complex system of symbols called "language."

During the last ten to fifteen years, the importance of the development during earliest years has been recognized. More and more studies show that what happens during a baby's early development greatly affects development in later life. Burton White, a leading authority on infant development, states in his book, *The First Three Years of Life*:

> *After seventeen years of research on how humans acquire their abilities, I have become convinced that it is to the first three years of life that we should now turn most of our attention. My own studies, as well as the work of many others, have clearly indicated that the experiences of those first years are far more important than we had previously thought. In their simple everyday activities, infants and toddlers form the foundations of all later development . . . To begin to look at a child's educational development when he or she is two years of age is already much too late. . . (Revised Edition, p. v & p. 5)*

This chapter divides development in the first three years into four phases. This division is intended merely to show a developmental sequence and not to imply fixed standards. The phases are: 1) birth to eight months, 2) eight to fourteen months, 3) fourteen to twenty-four months, and 4) twenty-four to thirty-six months.

Figure 1 presents developmental milestones in each major area of growth. It does not specify an age for each skill, but places the skill in the developmental phase in which it usually occurs. There is a very wide span of time for "normal" development, and your baby with Down syndrome may experience a sequence different from other children. Use the chart and the section that follows as an overview of development, a general road map. Later, this chapter reviews the conditions babies with Down syndrome may have that can impede their development.

Birth to Eight Months. During a baby's first eight months of life, coping with life outside the womb and gaining the rudiments of self-awareness are the major developmental goals. The skills she will learn are very basic, but very important: getting adjusted to sight, sound, touch, smell, taste, and becoming more interactive and mobile.

This is a time for laying foundations. Establishing love, security, and trust all help motivate babies to move, explore, and challenge themselves. Motivation itself is vital; this is a period to encourage curiosity and exploration, and to provide new experiences. During this period babies begin to learn the most fundamental aspects of life and their relationship to the world around them: that objects have weight and size, that people look and sound different, that things placed in mouths have a taste and a feel, that they themselves can bring about change. Parents can play a key role in identifying what interests their baby and in fostering those interests.

What skills emerge in the first eight months? A baby learns to roll, sit, and crawl; to respond to visual images and sound; to manipulate objects; and to relate to different people. She gains some control over her movements, begins to watch and listen, and practices new behaviors. By approximately eight months, when your baby can sit, reach for and hold a toy, and then hand it to you, she has learned an extraordinary number of skills. She has left her primitive reflexes behind, has begun to control her body movements, and is aware of herself in relation to others.

Eight to Fourteen Months. Some experts consider this a period of transition. Babies change from passive observers to purposeful doers. The changes that occur at this age are among the most critical in your baby's life. The three major developmental changes that occur during this period are: 1) the start of independent movement; 2) the first understanding of cause and effect and object permanence; and 3) the beginning use of language. From eight to fourteen months the ability to move brings about new freedom for exploration. Crawling, climbing, pulling to stand, cruising, and walking are practiced over and over. Refined hand skills will allow your child to pick up and explore small objects with her thumb and forefinger (pincer grasp), to use her hands in tandem to manipulate objects, and to begin to use objects like crayons, hammers, and spoons as tools.

These new motor skills are accompanied by major changes in cognitive ability. The twelve-month-old understands the concept of object permanence; this represents a quantum leap in reasoning ability. Research shows that the understanding of object permanence is closely related to a child's ability to use language. Both are abstract processes. These two skills naturally develop simultaneously. During this period, children dramatically increase their ability to understand words (receptive language), and begin to associate specific combinations of sounds with people, food, and objects in their world. Using words (expressive language) begins shortly after.

It is during this time that the strongest social bonds are established, usually to mother and father. Through these relationships your child learns the first do's and don't's of the family. The first inkling of independence also emerges, as she becomes able to play alone for short periods of time. She will also begin to help take care of herself. She will want to drink from a cup and try to feed herself with a spoon. This is the beginning of your child's ability to control her own needs.

Fourteen to Twenty-Four Months. The skills acquired during the first fourteen months launch the toddler into a

Figure 1. Developmental Milestones

	PHASE I: 0-8 MONTHS	PHASE II: 8-14 MONTHS
Gross Motor	• head control • turns over • sits • crawls	• pulls to stand • cruises • lowers self from standing position • walks alone • climbs upstairs
Fine Motor	• looks at hands • follows with eyes 180° • brings hands together • reaches • explores objects with hands • transfers objects hand to hand	• pincer grasp • scribbles • pushes toys • pokes at objects • one hand helps other
Language	• listens to sounds • turns to sound • babbles • laughs • responds to own name • makes vowel sounds	• recognizes names of common objects • enjoys listening to music • first words spoken
Cognitive	• looks from one object to another • looks after fallen object • pulls string to get object • uncovers toy he has seen hidden	• imitates use of toy • finds hidden toy (emergence of memory) • begins demonstrating cause and effect
Self Help	• reaches for bottle • finger feeds • holds bottle • drinks from cup with help	• drinks from cup with spilling • attempts spoon feeding • takes off socks
Social	• social smile • reaches for familiar person • smiles at mirror image • repeats performance laughed at	• understands "no" • cries when parent leaves • can play alone short periods • understands parent as resource

PHASE III: 14-24 MONTHS	PHASE IV: 24-36 MONTHS
• stoops and recovers • climbs into chairs • stands on one foot • walks up/down stairs holding on • kicks/throws ball • rides mobility toy	• runs, climbs • jumps in place • pulls wagon • rides tricycle
• builds tower of cubes • completes simple puzzles • turns pages of book • turns knobs	• strings beads • works latches and hooks • turns pages of book singularly • snips with scissors
• uses jargon • expands vocabulary • uses some phrases • names pictures • follows simple directions	• names body parts • uses some adjectives (color, size) • asks questions • understands some prepositions
• uses objects as tools • fits related objects together • uses trial and error • can arrange objects by size	• ability to use abstractions • draws recognizable face • understands "1", "2" • names common color • makes associations
• drinks from cup independently • combs hair • uses spoon independently • unzips • removes some clothes • partially toilet trained	• can put toys away • anticipates daily activities • pours • unties and removes shoes • puts on some clothes • toilet trained
• uses dramatic play/pretend • wants to be near other children • parallel play • negativism	• expands imaginary role play • shows sense of ownership • can wait turn • can ask for help • works problems out with less action, more reasoning

period of intense skill development for the next ten months. During this part of the second year, the ability to use language seems to explode. Spoken language changes from nonsensical babble to single words and then to phrases. The two-year-old can follow simple directions and likes to have stories read to her. The establishment of language enables her to communicate her ideas and feelings to others and to gather information. With this new use of language, your child moves to a much higher level of cognition, as well as into a real sense of personhood.

For the child approaching her second birthday, the world can be an exciting place. Everything is subject to observation and manipulation. All objects are explored in every possible way: feeling, tasting, smelling, poking, throwing. During this period, the testing will gradually shift from analysis to use.

This is a time for solving problems and playing with puzzles. Not only can blocks be stacked; they can be made into a house or fort. The hand skills that were recently established are now put to practice as your child begins to create and build. She is also able to help feed herself. These new hand skills open new arenas, both for practical and creative uses.

Socially, this is not an easy period for parent or child. During these months, the child struggles with the pushes and pulls of budding independence. Negativism may abound. She may oppose your wishes and directions; what you like, she may instantly dislike. This period is marked by your child's desire to assert her will and assume a new level of identity and independence. But it is also a time to explore the world of people. Although she may not yet play interactively, she will want to be near other children, either pursuing her own interests or engaging in the same activity. This stage is known as parallel play.

Twenty-Four to Thirty-Six Months. The skills acquired during this phase of development move the child to a dramatic new level of competence. The three-year-old has mastered most of the elementary gross motor skills. Walking has accelerated to running. Climbing and jumping are established in the motor repertoire. Fine motor, language, and cognitive skills are all expanded and refined. They are now demonstrated in more complex, creative, and constructive behaviors. Simple dramatic play now emerges as these complex skills are integrated.

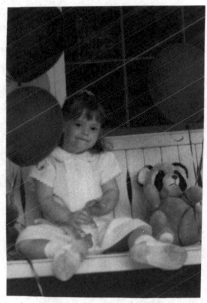

The child is able to envision herself in the place of another—to imagine, to make believe. Thought is no longer tied to concrete objects. Problem solving can take place by observation and reasoning. The child no longer needs to touch and feel an object in order to learn about it. She can look at an object, remember those she has played with before, and make decisions based on the objects she remembers. For example, your child may see a ball roll and therefore conclude that an orange will roll, too. In short, the three-year-old can reason and remember. She also has the ability to make associations, such as shoes and socks and rain and umbrellas, and to anticipate the consequences of her actions.

The social competence of three-year-olds is far more sophisticated. Toilet training occurs. They seek approval in a more dramatic way, and are able to use adults as resources. You will find it fun when your child comes and asks for the tool she needs to complete a project. Peers become much more important. During this period the child can be a successful part of a small group of two or three other children. Also during this period children can be quite competitive. It is in this environment that children learn the contrasting roles of leader and follower.

The first three years of life are marked by tremendous growth and development—from absolute dependence to semi-independence. Skills build upon each other so quickly that parents have a hard time keeping track of just what their child is capable of doing at any given time. Parents can only look back and remember when their child—now dressed and ready for nursery school—was utterly reliant on them and on her own instinctive reflexes for survival.

Expectations and Development

Parents of babies with Down syndrome, as well as parents of "normal" children, always want to know how their child will develop compared to other children. First, there is a very wide range of what is considered "normal" development. Some babies crawl at six months; others not until ten months; some skip crawling altogether. Each case is "normal." Your baby with Down syndrome may be within the normal range in some areas;

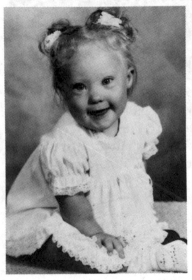

in others she may be slower than "normal." Your child may learn to walk sooner than some other children, while she may learn to talk later.

There is far more to development than how quickly your baby develops or how many skills she possesses. Quality, not quantity, is what is important. You should be more concerned that your daughter walks, integrating all of the component parts (well developed balance, equilibrium, bilateral coordination, posture, and strength), than that she walks early. Remember, each skill is a building block and a strong foundation is necessary. You can be one of the most important resources for building these good foundations. Therapeutic programs may also be an important partner in providing opportunities to develop these skills.

Babies with Down syndrome should be encouraged to explore, learn, and be curious, as all children should. If you step in too often with an answer or offer only little encouragement, development is hindered. Let your baby take risks. You may need to comfort your child when she falls trying to climb, but that is far easier than it is to stimulate an unmotivated child. Facilitation, the key word, means helping your child perform a skill *and* letting her do it herself.

The Development of Your Baby with Down Syndrome

We have presented a general sequence of development for the first three years of life. All children will learn skills in each of the six areas of development; their rate and sequence, however, will vary. A child's individual traits will determine her pattern. Some children take longer than others; some children don't master certain skills as well as others. The same is true of babies with Down syndrome.

All children have preferred ways of learning. For example, one child may learn best when a skill is demonstrated, while another may learn best using trial and error. Most will choose to learn new tasks in the way that is easiest for them. Because of the unique characteristics of babies with Down syndrome, they often need special guidance to help them master the same skills other babies acquire. You may need to discourage your child from taking the path of least resistance. For example, your baby may completely finish a bottle that is propped for her, but would do better if you encouraged her to hold the bottle with both hands herself. Doing this may involve a great deal of intervention initially, but will be rewarded in both fine and gross motor progress.

If you are aware of your baby's strengths and weaknesses you will be better able to give her the help she may need to develop optimally. If you know the stumbling blocks, you have a better chance of devising ways to overcome or minimize them. Children with Down syndrome can have specific characteristics that hinder development. This section reviews these traits.

Low Muscle Tone

Low muscle tone, or hypotonia, is very common in babies with Down syndrome. Their muscles feel floppy and flaccid. Although the degree of low tone varies from child to child, it generally affects all the baby's muscles.

How does low muscle tone affect development? The short answer is that its effects are quite extensive, but can be reduced with work. In addition, the effects usually diminish with age. As a newborn, your baby may move less. Her posture may be unusual. For example, when lying on her back, her legs may be wide apart and turned (rotated) out. Low muscle tone may contribute to delays in achieving major motor skills. Because muscles are floppier, attainment of head control, sitting, standing, and walking can be delayed and can also be less coordinated.

The earlier you begin to work to improve your baby's muscle tone the better. Seek the help of an infant specialist or physical or occupational therapist, if one is available. Techniques to increase muscle tone can begin within the first weeks of life. Intervention directed at improving muscle tone will improve the quality of your baby's motor and language skills. For example, low tone affects tongue and facial muscle control. By improving tone in these areas, your child will have the correct springboard for language development as well as improved appearance. Everyday routines can be altered to make a difference. You may be taught how to hold your baby in a more beneficial way. If your baby's legs tend to rotate out, it would be more beneficial to hold her with her legs facing forward and held together. Techniques like these can be easily incorporated in your daily routine and they can make a difference in your child's overall development.

Low muscle tone may also affect the development of both feeding and language skills. The same muscles we eat with are the muscles we use for speaking. When a child eats or talks, she uses muscles in her face, mouth, shoulders, and trunk. Poor muscle tone may make it difficult to form words or to move food around the mouth. Hypotonia throughout the trunk may also make it harder to produce the breath support necessary for spoken words. Early intervention will focus on eating and breathing patterns and how they are developing so as to maximize the skills needed for language.

Remember, a professional—a teacher or a therapist—can help you devise a plan to minimize the effects of the hypotonia. It is important to get professional help if possible because every baby is different. The amount of low tone itself varies from baby to baby, and how it may affect your baby in particular can vary as well. Children can have lower tone in certain parts of their body than others. That is why parents need instruction on working with low tone using techniques specifically tailored to their baby's needs.

Joint Flexibility

When joints are extraordinarily flexible, they are called hyperextensible. You may notice that your baby's hips and legs are easily rotated outward or that your baby can bend at the waist more easily than other babies. For example, you may notice that your child can fall asleep with her head on her own lap. This flexibility, which is closely related to low muscle tone, also affects motor development. If you are aware of this excessive joint flexibility, you can provide the extra support your baby needs. In the case of your sleeping baby, place a support, such as a rolled towel, in her lap to change her posture. You may also purchase foam triangles to be used while your child is sitting or sleeping.

Hyperextensible joints affect development by reducing the stability of your baby's limbs. In order to sit, crawl, and walk, your baby needs a stable foundation. Flexible joints and low muscle tone make these skills somewhat harder to achieve. Parents, however, can do much to help: something as simple as a firm hold on the hips as your child learns to pull up to a stand, or holding your baby's hips rather than her hands as she learns to walk can be of invaluable benefit. Professional input will, again, be helpful. The input of an infant specialist, occupational therapist, and physical therapist will include interventions to minimize the impact of joint flexibility.

Low Stamina

Babies with Down syndrome may have low stamina for physical tasks. This can be caused by a heart problem or sometimes by low muscle tone (or both). You can recognize low stamina if your baby seems to tire after simple activities. She may only be able to lift her head, push up on her forearms, grasp toys, pull up to a stand, or walk for short periods of time. Muscle strength can be improved, but stamina may take longer. Intervention over a long period of time, very much like a general fitness program, will help. Give your baby opportunities to use her muscles in a gradual program. Gentle "roughhousing" will help. Incorporate it into playtime. Hand strength can be improved by squeezing a sponge during bath time; arms can be strengthened by something as simple as pushing a toy. You want your baby to practice these activities during all the usual baby activities, such as dressing, changing diapers, bathing, and feeding. She may just need a little extra motivation and direction because these things may be more difficult for her. Exercises when well planned can serve as play as well as therapy.

In all of these areas—low muscle tone, joint flexibility, and low stamina—the effort to minimize their severity and impact is critical because they can slow motor development and diminish the quality of a skill. Motor development affects progress in every other developmental area. If your baby can't sit, she can't see the world clearly. If she can't sit with stability, she can't really use her hands. Clearly, the work to improve your baby's muscles and joints is critical and well worth the effort.

Tactile Sensitivity

Your baby's ability to integrate the sensations of touch, texture, and temperature may also be impaired. She may sometimes overreact to sensations, and this can cause developmental problems. Oversensitivity to touch (known as *tactile defensiveness*) occurs in children with Down syndrome, and when it does can interfere with your child's exploration of the world, with feeding, and with routine handling. Intervention programs generally address these problems by incorporating sensory integration techniques in their programs.

Hearing Loss

Many children with Down syndrome have some form of hearing loss. Chapter 3 discusses causes, treatments, and incidence of hearing loss. The percentages stated there are high enough to cause concern: Slightly less than half the children tested were found to have at least a mild hearing loss.

The effect of hearing loss on language development is great. Children who hear less, talk less and form sounds and words less accurately. They are unable to build their language skills without hearing speech. Because hearing is so vital to development of language, cognition, self-help, and social skills, it must be checked early. With early treatment—using antibiotics, ear tubes, or hearing aids—this potentially major stumbling block can be avoided.

Mental Retardation

In the past, all babies with Down syndrome were considered "severely and hopelessly" mentally retarded. Not so. Yes, children with Down syndrome have some degree of mental retardation. We often fail to remember, however, that mental retardation affects people very differently. The fact is that the majority of children with Down syndrome function in the mild to moderate range of mental retardation. Mental retardation means that your child will learn more slowly, not that she cannot learn.

What effect does mental retardation have on development? As with all factors affecting development, the severity of the problem determines the impact. Mental retardation does mean that progress in some areas will be slower. The ability to observe, analyze, and deal with abstract concepts is affected by cognitive ability. Skills that require your child to visualize objects or events she has not actually seen before may be difficult for her. For example, your child may repeat songs and rhythms she has been taught, but may have more trouble writing an original song on her own. Mental retardation can also cause your baby to have a shorter attention span and lower motivation than other babies. Both of these characteristics need to be addressed to help her learn.

Like other stumbling blocks, mental retardation can be addressed through intervention and its effects can be reduced. You should consult with teachers, arriving at a specific plan to facilitate your child's development. By breaking down tasks and concepts into smaller steps, difficult skills can be mastered. Hard work will pay off. Progress breeds more progress, along with a sense of accomplishment and pride in your child.

Your child will try hard to perform the desired task if it is presented to her in ways she can handle. For example, object permanence can be learned gradually, by providing repeated opportunities to experience it. Peek-a-boo or other games accomplish this goal in ways that are fun. Concepts are best taught initially with concrete objects that can be touched, seen, and explored rather than with pictures or words. Number concepts are made easier to learn when the objects counted are meaningful, such as cookies, body parts, and clothes. It is important to monitor your baby's attention span and motivation. New skills need to be practiced in short lesson periods and with a greater number of trials over time. A long lesson may not work well for your child. Again, your baby's teacher can work with you to design a complete individual plan for your child.

The coordination of several skills or a series of skills may be difficult for your baby with Down syndrome. For example, learning to use a form box or a shape puzzle will require breaking the task into its different parts (grasping, holding, and putting each piece in place). Over time, however, your baby will learn to combine these separate tasks into one enjoyable challenge. For example, your child may become an expert at jigsaw puzzles from playing with puzzles during her childhood.

Parents of babies with Down syndrome often worry about their child's IQ. Skill development, not scores on an intelligence test, should be the goal. IQ scores do not represent your child. There are many children who function much higher than a test score would indicate. IQ tests are designed to measure skills needed for academic success. Your child may have strengths in other areas, such as mechanical ability or interpersonal relationships which are not measured by these tests. Recent developments in the field of education have caused us to look differently at the concept of intelligence and to define it more broadly. Motivation, pride, security, determination, and love cannot be measured on an IQ test. Focus on your child, not on an IQ score.

Language Development

Infants with Down Syndrome also often have delays in speech and language development during the first several years of life. These delays can be the result of hearing loss, low muscle tone in the mouth and tongue, and the effect of Down syndrome on your child's cognitive development. Intervention can help a great deal to encourage your child's language development, and there are many good approaches to incorporating language goals into your daily interactions with your child. In later months, total communication techniques (combination of speech and manual signs) can also help your child's language development.

Helping Your Child's Development

Although this chapter has pointed out areas of delay in your baby's development, remember that these do not have to be barriers to learning and growing. Some areas of delay will be overcome; others will need to be circumvented. For example, although your child will learn to walk and run, she may have difficulty mastering a two-wheeled bike. This barrier can be circumvented by using training wheels or a large three-wheeled bike. Your goal is to maximize strengths and minimize weaknesses so that your child will realize her fullest potential.

Your hard work and your knowledge of your own baby's development will be rewarded. Studies show that babies with Down syndrome can develop quite well. Figure 2 shows one

Figure 2. Down Syndrome Development Compared to "Normal" Development

	CHILDREN WITH DOWN SYNDROME		"NORMAL" CHILDREN	
	Average	Range	Average	Range
smiling	2 months	1½ to 4 months	1 month	½ to 3 months
rolling over	8 months	4 to 22 months	5 months	2 to 10 months
sitting alone	10 months	6 to 28 months	7 months	5 to 9 months
crawling	12 months	7 to 21 months	8 months	6 to 11 months
creeping	15 months	9 to 27 months	10 months	7 to 13 months
standing	20 months	11 to 42 months	11 months	8 to 16 months
walking	24 months	12 to 65 months	13 months	8 to 18 months
talking, words	16 months	9 to 31 months	10 months	6 to 14 months
talking, sentences	28 months	18 to 96 months	21 months	14 to 32 months

(Pueschel, 1978)

study's findings of when babies with Down syndrome generally learn skills, compared with "normal" development.

Other studies show that early intervention—working to enhance your baby's development and overcome developmental delays —pays enormous dividends. Marci Hanson of the University of Oregon compared the development of babies with Down syndrome who were part of a program of early intervention with those who were not. The results speak for themselves. As Figure 3 illustrates, some of the children with Down syndrome who were involved in intervention programs developed faster than even the average "normal" child! But most dramatic is the difference between children with Down syndrome who were part of an early intervention program and those who did not participate.

Where to Get Developmental Help for Your Child

Parents can receive help with their baby's development from public or private sources. Under federal law, states are required to provide early intervention services to infants with disabilities from birth to age three. After age three, other federal laws require states to provide appropriate special education services. In these programs—detailed in Chapters 7 and 8—babies receive early intervention aimed at maximizing their potential.

Figure 3. Developmental Milestones

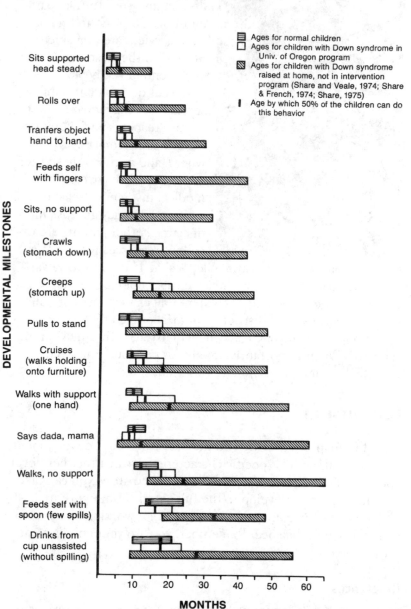

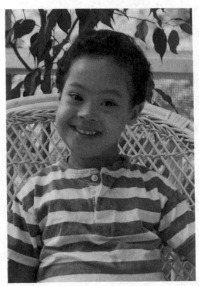

Check with your local school district and your state department of education to find out what services are available. Start with the Resource Guide at the end of the book.

What do you do if public services are inadequate? First, private teachers and therapists are available almost everywhere, and at times these therapy services are covered by medical insurance. Local organizations, advocacy groups, and, of course, other parents are excellent resources for information on what services are available locally. There is a wide variety of alternative arrangements, such as cooperative nursery schools and private group developmental classes. Ask for help: from your local school district, your local office of The Arc, advocacy groups, and anyone else who will listen, including your local media. Most importantly, do not let precious time go by; work with your child as much as you can.

Conclusion

This chapter has reviewed the basics of infant development, and how your child's specific characteristics can affect her development. Along the way, we have mentioned steps you can take to help your child develop to the full extent of her potential. There is, of course, more to parenting than working on development. Strive for balance. Remember, you are your child's greatest resource.

References

Aparicio, M. "Modelling and Early Language Acquisitions in Down's Syndrome." *Early Child Development and Care.* Vol. 44, March 1989, 51–59.

Carter, S. "The Other Side of the Story." *Exceptional Parent*. Vol. 9, No. 4, May-June 1989, 48–51.

Connolly, B., Morgan, S., Russell, F. "Evaluation of Children with Down Syndrome Who Participated in an Early Intervention Program. Second Follow-Up Study." *Physical Therapy*. Vol. 64, No. 10, October 1984, 1515–1519.

Dmitriev, V. "Cognition and the Acceleration and Maintenance of Developmental Gains among Children with Down Syndrome: Longitudinal Data." *Down's Syndrome Papers and Abstracts for Professionals*. Vol. 11, No. 1, January 1988, 6–11.

Hanson, M., Schwarz, R. "Results of a Longitudinal Intervention Program for Down's Syndrome Infants and Their Families." *Education and Training of the Mentally Retarded*. Vol. 13, No. 4, December 1978, 403–407.

Naganuma, G. "Early Intervention for Infants with Down Syndrome: Efficacy Research." *Physical and Occupational Therapy in Pediatrics*. Vol. 7, No. 1, Spring 1987, 81–92.

Oelwein, P., Fewell, R., Pruess, J. "The Efficacy of Intervention at Outreach Sites of the Program for Children with Down Syndrome and Other Developmental Disabilities." *Topics in Early Childhood Special Education*. Vol. 5, No. 2, Summer 1985, 78–87.

Pruess, J., et. al. "Language Development in Children with Down's Syndrome: An Overview of Recent Research." *Education and Training in Mental Retardation*. Vol. 22, No. 1, March 1987, 44–55.

Sloper, P., Glenn, S., Cunningham, C. "The Effect of Intensity Training on Sensori-Motor Development in Infants with Down's Syndrome." *Journal of Mental Deficiency Research*. Vol. 30, No. 2, June 1986, 149–162.

Tingey, C., Mortensen, L., Matheson, P., Doret, W. "Developmental Attainment of Infants and Young Children with Down Syndrome." *International Journal of Disability, Development, and Education*. Vol. 38, No. 1, 1991, 15–26.

Turkington, C. "Special Talents." *Psychology Today*. Vol. 21, No. 9, September 1987, 42–46.

Parent Statements

I thought there would be a whole lot of things a kid with Down syndrome couldn't do. But he does basically the same things other kids do. It just takes him longer to get there.

I guess the hardest part was waiting for her to roll over, waiting for her to crawl, waiting for her to sit up, waiting for her to walk.

I think I had an advantage because I didn't have anyone close to me who had a baby her age, so I wasn't constantly comparing her with anyone. Originally I had this picture in my mind of my baby being a super achiever—doing everything three months early. So it was kind of hard to wait for her to do things.

~ ᵕ ᵔ ᵕ ᵔ ᵕ ᵔ ᵕ ᵔ ᵕ ᵔ

Starting at birth, our county early intervention program provides all kinds of physical therapy to help with gross motor development. But the program is really reluctant to provide speech therapy to infants and toddlers, and doesn't even have enough speech therapists to go around. This seems really cockeyed. Every adult with Down syndrome I've ever met can walk, climb steps, tie his shoelaces, etc., quite adequately. But none of them even approaches "normalcy" in their speech. People with Down syndrome seem to have enormous trouble speaking fluently and articulating words correctly. *That's* the area of development I'm most concerned about.

~ ᵕ ᵔ ᵕ ᵔ ᵕ ᵔ ᵕ ᵔ ᵕ ᵔ

He has developed exactly like a normal child. It's just that his pace is slower. He's just like any child—he disobeys like another child, and he wants all the things that other little children want.

~ ᵕ ᵔ ᵕ ᵔ ᵕ ᵔ ᵕ ᵔ ᵕ ᵔ

There really is a wide range of capabilities among kids. You can't know. You can only provide the best kind of stimulation that you can as a parent, and deal with what is there genetically.

~ ᵕ ᵔ ᵕ ᵔ ᵕ ᵔ ᵕ ᵔ ᵕ

After you've gotten over the shock of finding out that your child has Down syndrome, you still have to wait around and see whether he's going to be "high functioning" or "low functioning" or somewhere in between. I worry a lot about that right now. Every time I see a kid with Down syndrome who is around the same age as my daughter, I watch him very closely to see whether he can do things my daughter can't. If he can't—if my daughter can do more things—I always feel happy. I know that sounds mean spirited, but I'm just looking for signs that my daughter may be a "high functioning" kid with Down syndrome.

With a normal child you just expect the development to happen, but with Chris every milestone is a great success. When he crawls or feeds himself with a spoon we're very happy, and we tell everyone about his progress. Other people might think we're going overboard, but we're very proud of every small victory.

I don't feel anxious about her development right now, but sometimes I wonder what it's going to be like when it's time for first grade, or when she's thirteen and on a fifth grade level. I think about that sometimes, but I try not to spend a lot of time worrying about it, because I really don't know how she'll do. She's doing pretty well now; I hope she'll keep it up.

I worry that my daughter might be smart enough to know that she's different, but not smart enough to truly be accepted by other kids. Maybe she will realize that people are laughing at her, but not understand why. Or maybe other kids will reject her when she tries to play with them, and she won't understand why. I'm torn. On the one hand, I want her to turn out to have really great cognitive skills. But on the other hand, I don't want her to be unhappy because she can almost, but not quite, do what other kids can do.

A new parent might wonder, "Will he smile? Will he hug me? Will he play? Will he recognize me?" From our experience, that's not something to worry about. You may feel a little frustrated when he doesn't do what Johnny next door is doing, but you'll find over time that he just reaches those stages a little later, but he'll reach them just the same. The big question after the first three years is "Will he keep up?" My feeling is that his horizons are unlimited. Quite realistically, I don't expect him to be a nuclear physicist, but I do hold out hopes for him to be independent and have a fulfilling life. I think any parent can be happy with that.

I can't say enough about how important it is for parents to know about normal development. You need to know how a child gets into a sitting position to help your child. Otherwise when you plop them down to sit, and they have their legs widespread, you're doing more harm than good. That's why early intervention is just crucial. Also, what comes next? You may see your child starting to do something and not realize it's a move toward the next step, particularly if it's your first child.

I think you have to be careful not to blame every problem with your child's development on Down syndrome. For example, our eighteen-month-old daughter was having trouble learning to feed herself with a spoon. The OT said it was because she had "poor separation" of the top lip from her tongue. But I think the real reason was that up until then, we almost never let her try to feed herself because we didn't want to deal with the mess. We hadn't given her the practice she needed.

There aren't guarantees for any child. Even if somebody is born with a normal set of chromosomes or perfect health, you don't know what's going to happen to that person. They could get sick, or they could grow up perfectly healthy but have some inability to cope with life. There are a lot of people in the world who have normal capabilities but don't know how to use them or who use them for bad purposes.

~ ~ ~ ~ ~ ~ ~ ~ ~ ~ ~

I still have an unbelievable consciousness of her needs. I know where she is in all areas. But I don't think it's that hard to do. You need to have fun with your child and talk to her, whether you're alone with her or just driving to school.

~ ~ ~ ~ ~ ~ ~ ~ ~ ~ ~

I used to go to school with her one day a week and come home and feel that I had to push because I wasn't seeing progress in this or that area. I often thought Laurie would never count to ten, and now she can go well beyond that. It can get frustrating when teachers and therapists are reminding you over and over of the things you need to do, and you don't see change from one week to the next. But you're not going to see changes every week, especially when you're monitoring it almost too closely.

~ ~ ~ ~ ~ ~ ~ ~ ~ ~ ~

Sometimes he won't seem to progress at all for several months and then all of a sudden he'll take off like a rocket, and the progress is extremely noticeable and a real thrill. In our other children, the plateaus are a lot shorter. When he does progress, it's more noticeable.

~ ~ ~ ~ ~ ~ ~ ~ ~ ~ ~

Besides having Down syndrome, my daughter was born six weeks prematurely as a twin. I'm never completely sure whether delays are due to the Down syndrome, the prematurity, or being a twin.

~ ~ ~ ~ ~ ~ ~ ~ ~ ~ ~

Sometimes people find that once they have a kid with special needs, they learn a lot about child development. It makes the bringing up of children later extremely interesting. I can watch Josh's younger brother for hours. It's so fascinating because of what I've learned from Josh about the learning process—how children learn gross motor skills, fine motor skills, speech. It has deepened our enjoyment of the baby because we know so much more about the process.

Seven

⌁⌁⌁⌁⌁

Teaching Your Baby with Down Syndrome: An Introduction to Early Intervention

Linda Diamond, M.S.*

What Is Early Intervention?

During the past fifteen years, many types of educational programs for babies, for parents, and for parents and babies together have been developed. This chapter examines a special type of educational program designed to aid the development of babies with Down syndrome. Early intervention differs from what you may hear referred to as "infant stimulation" or "infant stim." Interest in babies and infant development has prompted many groups to offer "stimulating" products, ideas, and classes. Of course, stimulating your baby is a good thing to do. But when a baby has special needs, the stimulation has to be special, too.

Early developmental intervention programs for children with special needs and their families can take many forms and

* Linda Diamond holds a Masters in Special Education and is an Infant Development Specialist and Family Coordinator in the early intervention program at the Ivymount School in Rockville, Maryland. She is also Intervention Coordinator for Pride in Parenting, a grant funded by NIH-DC Initiative to Reduce Infant Mortality.

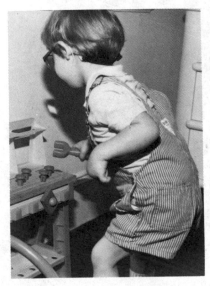

can include a wide variety of services. There are, however, many elements that are common to almost all early intervention programs. Thinking separately about "early," "developmental," and "intervention," will help you understand the purpose of these programs. "Early" usually refers to the age range of birth to three years. "Developmental" refers to the growth and development of your baby and to the continual acquisition of new skills. "Intervention" means planned, specific, conscious, and specialized ways of interacting with your baby to enhance his development. Together these elements form a program to help children who in some way are not developing like other children.

Because your baby has Down syndrome, his development will be different from that of other babies. Every baby is unique, possessing both strengths and weaknesses. However, as earlier chapters have explained, your baby is more likely to encounter certain developmental problems due to Down syndrome. Maybe he does not move his arms and legs vigorously; maybe he does not follow objects with his eyes or seems to be disinterested; perhaps feeding is more difficult and slower than it is for other babies. These things are not your fault or your baby's fault, but are examples of how Down syndrome can affect him.

Chapter 6 reviewed how the particular characteristics of Down syndrome affect development. But each baby is different. Learning how your baby's development is affected and how to best handle and interact with him to help him grow and develop is the major purpose of early intervention. For instance, if your child has low muscle tone, there are exercises that can help improve it. If your child seems unresponsive, there are many different types of interaction that can be tried to motivate him.

There are many ways of handling and interacting with babies. Some babies prefer certain kinds of handling to others. For example, some babies want and need cuddling while others would rather be placed comfortably in their crib with a mobile in sight. Your baby will also have preferences. His preferences, however, may not always work to his benefit. They might in fact work against his development. For example, your baby's preference to stiffen or "lock" his leg and hip joints as a way to stand can work against good development. Your early intervention program can show you how to minimize this and other tendencies through exercise and proper positioning.

Early intervention requires highly trained specialists who can work with you and your baby to maximize his early development. Early intervention is a process; it changes as your baby changes and as you and your baby's teachers learn what techniques work best for your baby. The other purpose of early intervention is to support you in your efforts to integrate your baby into your family in addition to teaching you specific techniques to use with your baby.

Early intervention can help your baby develop to the best possible level. This can be done through direct "hands on" intervention, but most importantly by helping you learn how to best help your baby. No one can predict precisely what the future holds for a baby with Down syndrome, and early intervention is not a magical cure, but working at development from early infancy is important in helping your baby reach his full potential.

People and Programs

Your child needs an early intervention program that is designed to meet his special needs. Early intervention programs can take many different forms and can include a wide variety of services and professionals. In addition, there are significant differences in the quality and quantity of programs in each state, county, and city. This section reviews the many types of early infant intervention programs and describes the various professionals who work with babies with Down syndrome.

Professionals

Depending on the specific programs in your area and on your baby's needs, you may work with one or all of the professionals described below. These professionals may work as a team in an early intervention program or may work individually to provide particular services in a private practice setting. In any case, they should be highly trained in their area of expertise and specifically experienced with babies with Down syndrome.

Developmental Pediatrician. A developmental pediatrician may be a part of the early intervention team. This doctor has specialized training in development combined with his or her medical education. If there is a developmental pediatrician on your team, he or she may review your child's records and consult with you and the team . He or she may also participate directly in assessments and planning for your child. He or she can give you a lot of information about how Down syndrome may be affecting your child. Although there are not many developmental pediatricians, there may be one in your community.

Infant Educator. An infant educator is a teacher trained to work on helping your baby's overall development, and specifically on his cognitive development. The teacher should be knowledgeable about typical development and about development that is not proceeding typically. The infant educator will focus his or her attention on your baby's responsiveness to stimulation (for example, following toys or objects with his eyes), on how he plays, on his social development, and on the development of his ability to understand concepts (for example, that hitting a large button on a musical toy will make it start playing). He or she will tailor his or her work with your baby to his age and level of development through infancy and toddlerhood.

The infant educator, along with other professionals, may also work with you on the daily care of your baby. The exact role of the infant educator varies greatly from program to program. In some programs, infant educators focus on parents and infants, while in others the emphasis is on the child alone. The actual work of an infant educator may look more like playing games with your child. For example, she may teach object permanence by playing a "peek-a-boo" game or by hiding a favorite toy and then helping your child to find it.

Pediatric Physical Therapist. A pediatric physical therapist will focus on your child's gross motor development. She will assess how your child moves, and will determine what movements are difficult for your baby. She is concerned with muscle tone, reflex development, movement patterns, stability, and motor development. She will assist your baby in using muscles effectively to move. The

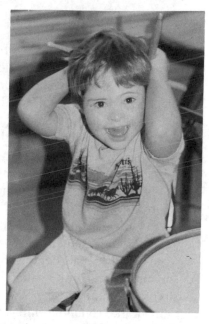

physical therapist's goal is to foster the best and most typical movement patterns for your baby. For example, she will work with your baby to learn how to get into a sitting position correctly by pushing up from a side-sitting position, rather than by spreading his legs and sitting straight up.

A physical therapist may work with your child once or twice a week. During these sessions, your baby will work very hard as the therapist uses a series of exercises to help him move. For example, the therapist will help teach your baby to roll onto his tummy by placing him on his side, bending his top leg, and gently moving him to give him the feeling of rolling onto his tummy.

The therapist may have specialized training in neurodevelopmental treatment (NDT), which is a comprehensive approach to pediatric physical therapy that emphasizes the subtle aspects of movements and posture. For example, when teaching your child to sit, an NDT therapist will look closely at the position of your baby's back, shoulders, hips, and legs rather than just if he is sitting. An NDT therapist focuses on the quality of your child's position and movements. Other professionals who work with your baby, such as occupational therapists, speech/language therapists, and infant educators, may also have this specialized training.

Pediatric Occupational Therapist. Occupational therapists are also trained to look at how babies move, but concentrate on the positions of shoulders, arms, and hands, and very importantly, on how this affects his ability to do activities that involve reaching for and holding objects. These therapists will work with your baby to improve his fine motor skills. For example, the therapist will play with your baby using different toys such as a toy telephone to encourage him to use his index finger. This therapist's work also includes assisting you in helping your baby develop self-help skills, such as dressing and washing, and even early skills like reaching for his bottle, grabbing a pacifier, or splashing in a bath.

The occupational therapist will also help your child with sensory processing, or how he takes in information through his senses of vision, hearing, touch, and movement. Sometimes babies do not like touching things that feel different, such as mushy, rough, or fuzzy objects. Because they learn so much from touching, however, it is important to help them feel comfortable with a variety of textures. The occupational therapist will help your child by gradually introducing him to a wide variety of objects and textures.

Pediatric Speech and Language Therapist. These therapists are trained to look at how your baby uses the muscles of his mouth and face to eat and to make sounds. This is called oral motor development. From early infancy, the speech therapist can be a resource for concerns or problems with feeding (such as refusing to take food from a spoon or refusing to eat food that is not completely smooth) and will work with you and your baby to solve them. For example, to overcome resistance to new foods, the therapist will use different types of touch to your baby's face and mouth to help prepare him for eating. In addition, this therapist will work with your baby to develop early communication skills, such as an understanding of language, use of gestures, and making sounds. Later he or she will focus on the proper articulation of sounds and words. This therapist can also evaluate your baby's responsiveness to sound and can help spot potential hearing problems.

Mental Health Professional. Some early intervention programs have counsellors, social workers, or other mental health professionals who can provide emotional support and counselling to families. Some issues to focus on include adjusting to having a baby with Down syndrome, what to say to other people, and how to balance your baby's needs with the needs of the rest of your family. At different times, families have found this to be a very helpful service; it can also be sought privately if not available through an intervention program. The service provider can be a social worker, psychologist, family counsellor, or a specially trained infant teacher. Often babies and parents are seen together as part of this service.

Your child's program may also sponsor a parent support group. This group might be led by the mental health professional, by a teacher, or by a parent. These groups offer support, information, counselling, and an opportunity to share problems with parents who have similar concerns. In addition to your child's early intervention program, many special interest organizations such as your local office of The Arc sponsor parent groups.

Pediatric Nurse. A nurse may be part of the early intervention program in your area, or may be available through your local health department, hospital, or visiting nurse association. He or she may assist with daily medical care and use of equipment (such as sleep apnea monitors, feeding tubes, and medications), and might also be a source of information about early development.

Case Manager. One member of your baby's early intervention team may serve as a case manager or coordinator. It is the case manager's job to gather information and ideas from the team working with you and your baby, and to coordinate the different services being provided. Often the case manager is the infant teacher, but any one of the other professionals may also fill this role. As the primary service provider, the case manager will be the one to give you an overall picture of your baby's development, to show you how each area of development interacts with

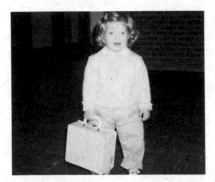

another, and to incorporate all of this information into your child's program.

You, however, are ultimately your baby's case manager. As you learn about his needs and about early intervention, you will become the coordinator of information about your baby; the professionals will become consultants as much as teachers to you. There is simply no substitute for direct parent involvement. You know your baby and your family best, and you are with your baby more than anyone else. Your baby's development goes on all the time and opportunities to enhance that development occur many times over the day. The professionals can make suggestions and work with your baby for the time they have, but you will be the best source for helping your baby and judging which recommendations work and which do not.

As you can see, there are many professionals who could work with your child. Each serves a different function and each has a specialty. It is possible that the team could include a different professional for each specialty, or one or two people who provide all of the services, or a combination of professionals working separately. Remember, there is great variety in the way services are provided in different locations. Check out your local programs; many different program models can work. Find caring professionals to help you obtain the services you and your baby need, especially in the first months after his birth.

Programs

Just as there are different professionals, organizations, and funding agencies who provide services, there are also many types of programs available for babies with Down syndrome. The following descriptions will help guide you in exploring the different programs available to you in many communities.

Family-Centered Service. This kind of program focuses on the family as a whole—parents and children together. Although your baby's special needs are the central focus, this program goes a little further. In addition to working with your baby, the program works with families to integrate the child and the special services he needs into the family. In a family approach, the staff would gear its work with a child to the family's overall circumstances. They would consider such things as family lifestyle, the parents' work schedules, other children, the family's daily routine, members of the extended family, the baby's health and care requirements, and how the program's recommendations fit into the family's life. By looking at this wide variety of factors, family-centered programs try to help both children and families as a single unit.

Child-Centered Service. This type of program is somewhat more traditional than a family-centered program, and far less common today than in the past. In it there is one "client"— the baby. The program usually consists of staff who provide specific suggestions to parents to help their child reach developmental goals. Family life, varying lifestyles, and other family members are not considered as strongly or to the same degree as a family-centered model. Under the Individuals with Disabilities Education Act (IDEA), early intervention services are now required to be family-centered, so this approach may disappear over time.

There is no one ideal program. All programs are really a collection of people with a common purpose. You will find that the quality and usefulness of a program depends to a great extent on the staff, the program goals, and how those match with your current needs. Try to find the type of program that works best for you and your baby.

Home-Based and Center-Based Programs

There are two places babies with Down syndrome receive early intervention services: at home or at a "center." Babies who have health problems such as heart defects require home care, while children with good health can be served at home or go to a center. This section reviews how early intervention programs work at home or at "school."

In home-based services, members of the early intervention team come to your home for regularly scheduled visits to work with you and your baby. They may all visit together once a week, or each may come separately. How many teachers or therapists visit and how often they visit can change as your baby's needs change. Home-based services are generally provided to babies up to three years of age. Home-based services are necessary for children who, because of fragile health, should not be exposed to other children, but other families may also find this program the best for their baby or toddler.

During a home visit the teacher or therapist will work with your baby, focusing on the different areas of development. Each area of development can involve different activities and exercises. For example, activities to improve gross motor development might include supporting your child in a sitting position while encouraging him to reach for a toy. Or it might include the therapist holding your baby on a big rubber ball and moving it into different positions to force him to exercise different muscles.

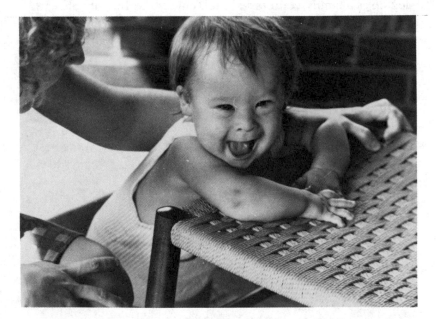

The teacher or therapist will likely want you to try the various activities with your child. He or she may work with you and your baby together, or just work with your baby, or perhaps have you do most of the work. The teacher will also ask questions about what you have been observing in your child between visits. Questions might include, "Have you seen your baby sit for a few seconds? Does your baby seem to prefer bright, shiny toys to noisy toys? Does your baby prefer to move around rather than sit and play?" Often, at the end of each session, the teacher or therapist will leave suggestions—frequently in writing—about things to try with your baby until the next visit.

In many programs, the teacher will bring a bag of toys and equipment to each session. He or she may leave some of these for you to use with your child or suggest ways to work with your child. For example, a favorite of physical therapists is a big rubber ball that can be used for abdominal exercises, developing balance, and many other motor skills.

Home visits are also a time for you to discuss problems and concerns. For example, if feeding is a problem or if your child's leg movements don't seem right, these can be discussed during a home visit. This exchange of information enables both you and the teacher to work on those areas that need the most help and to continually evaluate your child's progress.

Much of what goes on during a home visit also occurs in center-based programs. The major difference between home- and center-based programs is that in a center-based program you bring your baby to a "center," which could be a school, health department, or private office. The "classroom" might look like a typical classroom scaled to the size and needs of babies and toddlers. The center may also have additional rooms for physical therapy with heavy mats on the floor, mirrors, and other equipment.

Center-based programs may be individual, with just you, your baby, and the teacher or therapist, or may include small groups of parents and their babies along with the staff. In group programs, you may receive less individual attention, but you may learn different techniques from the other parents and children. In addition, your child will learn social skills from being around other children, such as noticing and playing near other children, learning to take turns, and sharing toys. In some cases, home- and center-based services are combined.

The services that your child receives through either home-based or center-based programming depends on what is in his Individualized Family Service Plan (IFSP). This plan is required by the IDEA. IFSPs describe your child's strengths and needs, your family's resources and concerns, and the early intervention services to be provided. This information is based primarily on your input, but will also come from a developmental evaluation of your child. In addition to the information you provide, it is also important to ask about the professionals' impressions of your child and what services you are entitled to under the law. The process works differently in different areas of the country.

Wherever you live, your priorities for your child and your family should be followed. In some instances this may be the only factor that guides the services your child receives. It is important that the priorities you identify be the central focus; however, other services that could be helpful to your child which you might not be aware of should also be explored. Many services that could help your family (such as respite care, family counselling, home health care) may be stipulated in the IFSP, but are not necessarily funded by the law.

Figure 1 shows sample IFSP forms.

The Evaluation

You may be referred to an early intervention program when you receive the diagnosis of Down syndrome. Some programs may start quickly with informal evaluations and initial recommendations, and then later schedule a more formal developmental evaluation. Each local education agency, school district, or state education agency will have a phone number to call to start the process of obtaining services. Ask your doctor, a teacher, your local school district, the local office of The Arc, and other parents of children with Down syndrome how to get in touch with the program serving your area.

Figure 1. Sample IFSP Forms (pages 193–201)

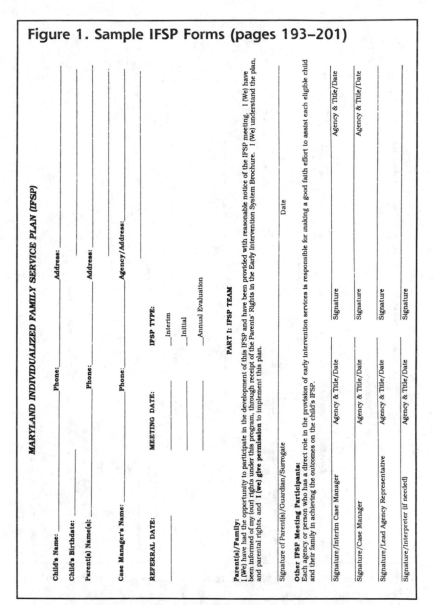

MARYLAND INDIVIDUALIZED FAMILY SERVICE PLAN (IFSP)

Child's Name: _____ Phone: _____ Address: _____

Child's Birthdate: _____

Parent(s) Name(s): _____ Phone: _____ Address: _____

Case Manager's Name: _____ Phone: _____ Agency/Address: _____

REFERRAL DATE: _____ MEETING DATE: _____ IFSP TYPE:

___ Interim
___ Initial
___ Annual Evaluation

PART I: IFSP TEAM

Parent(s)/Family:
I (We) have had the opportunity to participate in the development of this IFSP and have been provided with reasonable notice of the IFSP meeting. I (We) have been informed of my (our) rights under this program, through receipt of the Parents' Rights in the Early Intervention System Brochure. I (We) understand the plan, and parental rights, and **I (we) give permission** to implement this plan.

_____ _____
Signature of Parent(s)/Guardian/Surrogate Date

Other IFSP Meeting Participants:
Each agency or person who has a direct role in the provision of early intervention services is responsible for making a good faith effort to assist each eligible child and their family in achieving the outcomes on the child's IFSP.

Signature/Interim Case Manager	Signature	Agency & Title/Date
Agency & Title/Date		
Signature/Case Manager	Signature	Agency & Title/Date
Agency & Title/Date		
Signature/Lead Agency Representative	Signature	
Agency & Title/Date		
Signature/Interpreter (if needed)	Signature	
Agency & Title/Date		

The process will begin by your providing background information. This can be done by phone or in person with the staff of your local Infants and Toddlers Program. Most often, assessments will be scheduled to help determine your baby's needs for early intervention services. If a developmental evaluation has

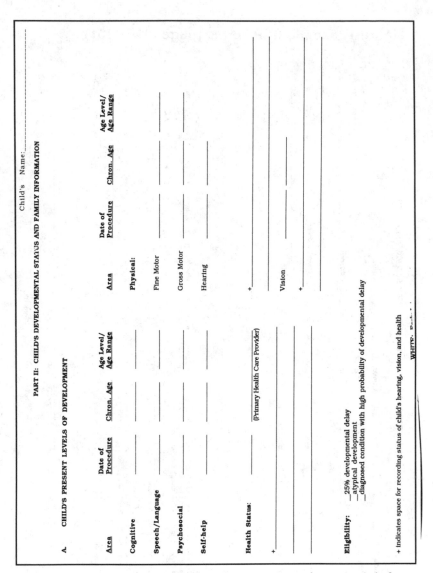

been completed recently, that report may contain enough information without doing a new evaluation.

Developmental evaluations can provide you with important information—sometimes new information, sometimes an objective confirmation of what you already know. The evaluation can tell you the areas of your child's development that are strong and the areas that are weak, so that an effective early interven-

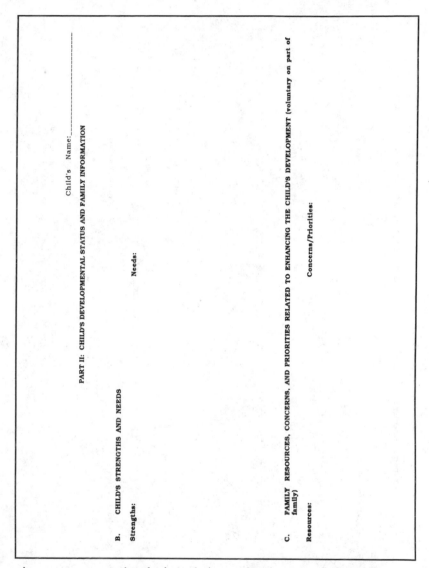

Child's Name:_____

PART II: CHILD'S DEVELOPMENTAL STATUS AND FAMILY INFORMATION

B. CHILD'S STRENGTHS AND NEEDS

Strengths:

Needs:

C. FAMILY RESOURCES, CONCERNS, AND PRIORITIES RELATED TO ENHANCING THE CHILD'S DEVELOPMENT (voluntary on part of family)

Resources:

Concerns/Priorities:

tion program can be designed. An evaluation can also give you an idea of how your baby's skills compare to other babies and enables you to monitor progress through check-up evaluations.

During an evaluation, your child will be given specific activities to do. Some of the activities will be easy for him and some will be hard; this is to identify your child's developmental strengths and weaknesses. The assessment could be performed

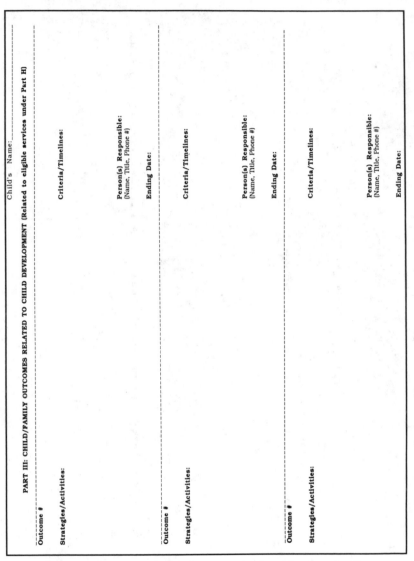

Child's Name: _____

PART III: CHILD/FAMILY OUTCOMES RELATED TO CHILD DEVELOPMENT (Related to eligible services under Part H)

Outcome #

Strategies/Activities:

Criteria/Timelines:

Person(s) Responsible:
(Name, Title, Phone #)

Ending Date:

Outcome #

Strategies/Activities:

Criteria/Timelines:

Person(s) Responsible:
(Name, Title, Phone #)

Ending Date:

Outcome #

Strategies/Activities:

Criteria/Timelines:

Person(s) Responsible:
(Name, Title, Phone #)

Ending Date:

by an early interventionist or by a team of professionals. Your baby's performance can provide crucial data, but it is also important for you to provide information about your baby to the person assessing him during the evaluation. If the evaluator does not see your baby regularly, he or she may not see everything your baby can do and may interpret your baby's performance differently than you would. That is why your observations about

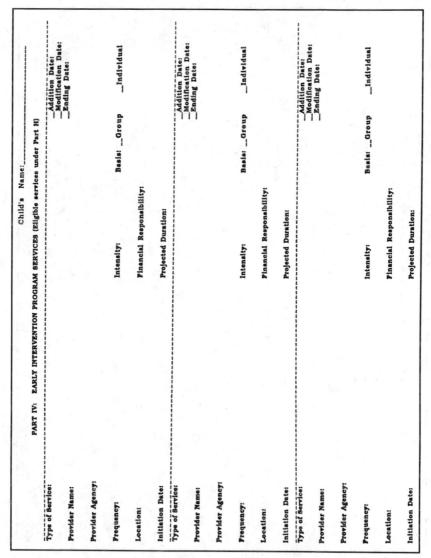

PART IV: EARLY INTERVENTION PROGRAM SERVICES (Eligble services under Part H)

Child's Name: _____

Type of Service: _____
Provider Name:
Provider Agency:
Frequency:
Location:
Initiation Date:

Intensity:
Financial Responsibility:
Projected Duration:

Basis: ___Group ___Individual

___Addition Date:
___Modification Date:
___Ending Date:

Type of Service: _____
Provider Name:
Provider Agency:
Frequency:
Location:
Initiation Date:

Intensity:
Financial Responsibility:
Projected Duration:

Basis: ___Group ___Individual

___Addition Date:
___Modification Date:
___Ending Date:

Type of Service: _____
Provider Name:
Provider Agency:
Frequency:
Location:
Initiation Date:

Intensity:
Financial Responsibility:
Projected Duration:

Basis: ___Group ___Individual

___Addition Date:
___Modification Date:
___Ending Date:

your child are so important. It can make a difference for the evaluator to know that your baby does things at home that he did not do at the evaluation, or vice versa. Results of the evaluation are usually given to you at the end of the assessment. This is a time for you to ask questions and share your impressions.

The evaluation will hopefully assist you in finding a good program for your child. If there is no appropriate infant program

Child's Name: _____

PART V: OTHER CHILD/FAMILY OUTCOMES (Related to non-required services under Part H)

Outcome #

Strategies/Activities:

Criteria/Timelines:

Person(s) Responsible:
(Name, Title, Phone #)

Ending Date:

Outcome #

Strategies/Activities:

Criteria/Timelines:

Person(s) Responsible:
(Name, Title, Phone #)

Ending Date:

Outcome #

Strategies/Activities:

Criteria/Timelines:

Person(s) Responsible:
(Name, Title, Phone #)

Ending Date:

in your area, developmental evaluations may be available through a particular hospital department, such as genetics, birth defects, neonatology, or physical medicine. For parents in areas without special infant programs, these hospital departments could provide contact with professionals knowledgeable about infant development and could be a good place to ask questions.

Child's Name: _____

PART VI: SERVICE LINKAGES FOR OTHER CHILD/FAMILY OUTCOMES (Non-required services under Part H)

Type of Service: _____

Primary Client: _____

Provider Agency: _____

Funding Source(s): _____

__Addition Date:
__Modification Date:
__Ending Date:

Type of Service: _____

Primary Client: _____

Provider Agency: _____

Funding Source(s): _____

__Addition Date:
__Modification Date:
__Ending Date:

Type of Service: _____

Primary Client: _____

Provider Agency: _____

Funding Source(s): _____

__Addition Date:
__Modification Date:
__Ending Date:

Type of Service: _____

Primary Client: _____

Provider Agency: _____

Funding Source(s): _____

__Addition Date:
__Modification Date:
__Ending Date:

Type of Service: _____

Primary Client: _____

Provider Agency: _____

Funding Source(s): _____

__Addition Date:
__Modification Date:
__Ending Date:

Type of Service: _____

Primary Client: _____

Provider Agency: _____

Funding Source(s): _____

__Addition Date:
__Modification Date:
__Ending Date:

Private pediatric therapists may also be available and able to provide needed services to you and your baby.

Several types of agencies may have early intervention programs under their auspices. In some areas there may be more than one source for early intervention; in others the resources may be more limited. Generally, services are offered through:

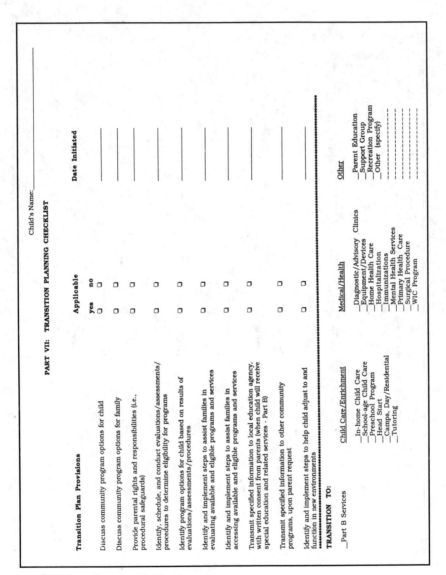

Child's Name: _____

PART VII: TRANSITION PLANNING CHECKLIST

Transition Plan Provisions	Applicable yes	no	Date Initiated
Discuss community program options for child	☐	☐	
Discuss community program options for family	☐	☐	
Provide parental rights and responsibilities (i.e., procedural safeguards)	☐	☐	
Identify, schedule, and conduct evaluations/assessments/ procedures to determine eligibility for programs	☐	☐	
Identify program options for child based on results of evaluations/assessments/procedures	☐	☐	
Identify and implement steps to assist families in evaluating available and eligible programs and services	☐	☐	
Identify and implement steps to assist families in accessing available and eligible programs and services	☐	☐	
Transmit specified information to local education agency, with written consent from parents (when child will receive special education and related services - Part B)	☐	☐	
Transmit specified information to other community programs, upon parent request	☐	☐	
Identify and implement steps to help child adjust to and function in new environments	☐	☐	

TRANSITION TO:

__Part B Services

Child Care/Enrichment
__In-home Child Care
__School-age Child Care
__Preschool Program
__Head Start
__Camps, Day/Residential
__Tutoring

Medical/Health
__Diagnostic/Advisory Clinics
__Equipment/Devices
__Home Health Care
__Hospitalization
__Immunizations
__Mental Health Services
__Primary Health Care
__Surgical Procedure
__WIC Program

Other
__Parent Education
__Support Group
__Recreation Program
__Other (specify)

1. Public school districts.

2. Private schools that serve children whose special requirements cannot be met by the public school district.

MARYLAND INFANTS AND TODDLERS DATA ADD/CHANGE FORM

Date Form Completed: _____

Child's Name: _____ Birthdate: _____

CHILD AND FAMILY INFORMATION

Child's Social Security #: _____ Child's Medical Assistance #: _____

Child's Address: _____ Child's Phone: # _____

Mother's Name: _____ Mother's Birthdate: _____ Mother's Social Security #: _____

Mother's Address: _____ Mother's Phone #: _____

Father's Name: _____

Father's Address: _____ Father's Phone #: _____

Other Family/Contact Name: _____ Relationship to Child: _____

Other Family/Contact Address: _____ Other Phone #: _____

CHILD STATUS

___ Inactive: ___ Inactive as of (date): _____

___ Deceased   ___ Out of county
___ No longer eligible   ___ Parent withdrawal
___ Not in Maryland   ___ Whereabouts unknown
___ Transition (Part B/Other)   ___ Other (Please specify) _____

INDIVIDUALIZED FAMILY SERVICE PLAN (IFSP) REVIEW

Review Date:	Review Type:	Review Status:	Case Manager :
	___ Six month	___ Continue IFSP	Name: _____
	___ Parent request	___ Modify IFSP	Agency: _____
	___ Provider request	___ End IFSP	Phone #: _____
	___ Parent/provider request		Signature: _____

___ I (We) have had the opportunity to participate in the review of this IFSP and approve the review status indicated above.
___ I (We) give permission to the early intervention program to implement attached outcome and service revisions.

Signature of Parent(s)/Guardian/Surrogate _____   Date _____

3. Private therapists (physical, occupational, and speech).

4. Regional children's hospitals.

5. Programs affiliated with universities and university hospitals.

6. State, county, or municipal health departments and divisions of mental retardation or developmental disabilities.

7. Local organizations such as The Arc and local Down syndrome groups.

If you have difficulty getting the information you need, your local chapter of The Arc, the local or state special education agency, or the local Down syndrome association may be able to steer you in the right direction. Use the Resource Guide at the end of this book to start your search. Other parents who are already receiving services for their children can also be most helpful.

In choosing a program it is important to obtain information about the programs in your area. Observe a program in operation, interview the staff, and talk to parents whose children are in the program. Then make your choice. You will then have to work with the professionals in the Infants and Toddlers Program to determine what services will be best. Remember, this field of infant development is new to you, and it is impossible for you to become an expert overnight. But no choice is permanent; if the program you pick does not meet your needs or your baby's needs, find an alternative by making changes with the staff or by choosing another program. In this process of choosing a program, the experience of other parents can be invaluable.

Parents as Teachers: The Parent-Professional Partnership

The essence of early intervention is direct parent involvement. Most programs stress the parents as the primary teacher of their baby. By contrast, in traditional education you may have heard that "parents should not be their children's teacher." But when it comes to teaching your baby with Down syndrome, your role is critical—especially because your baby is starting his education so early.

Parents know their babies best and have the greatest opportunity to work and play with them. Because babies constantly change and are largely unpredictable in how they respond on a particular day and time, playing with them in specific ways every day is important. In addition to the scheduled visits of the intervention team, special activities can be incorporated into your baby's daily routine. You will receive guidance about how to work with your child as you and he go through each day together. In order to do this you need a great deal of information. You cannot be expected to know automatically how to meet the special needs of your baby. You need to learn about the special handling techniques, observational skills, and teaching strategies. Early intervention teachers and therapists can give you this information.

You are the consumer of a very specialized and very personal service. Someone will not only help your baby to learn, but will also assist and guide you. Establishing a partnership with your early intervention professionals should be a very positive experience. Ideally, it is a two-way relationship. You can learn teaching techniques and hear about new ideas and information, and your child's teachers can learn from you about your baby and your family. For example, a special seat to support your baby and to encourage him to reach out for a toy may be a great idea, but because of your other children or the layout of your house this may not work for you. Or you may notice your baby trying to hold his head up; the teacher may suggest ways to strengthen neck muscles and new ways to motivate your baby. In a good working parent-professional relationship, both partners listen to each other and work together to develop ideas that work for you and your child.

The positive aspects of this type of relationship—such as the relief of having someone join you in helping your baby—can be a great help. On the other hand, this kind of service can feel very intrusive and sometimes can trigger feelings of inadequacy. You may feel that you are forced to share parenting with a professional whom you may see as competent and knowledgeable while you may feel incompetent and ignorant. Having someone come into your home to work with your baby may make you feel as though you are being taught something you should already know. Also, time—already a precious commodity—is further strained by having to fit in visits of the intervention team. The ups and downs just described are part and parcel of the parent-professional partnership. This pull and push is perfectly normal and is to be expected.

Here are some hints for making the parent-professional partnership work for you and your baby:

- There are still professionals with whom you may come into contact who view themselves as "experts" and who think you should be unquestioningly grateful for the help you are receiving. Never forget that this is your baby and you are the consumer of these services for both of you. Don't be bullied or intimidated.
- If you don't understand something about your child or the services he is receiving, ask questions. Discuss what is and is not working for you and your baby. Most of all, share your concerns.
- Take good care of yourselves. This means that the goals of the early intervention program should fit into your family's life. The reality of having many responsibilities is that, although the goals for your baby are extremely important, there are times when you cannot work toward them as you would like. This happens to everyone—and it is important to your family that you all have a balanced life.
- If you think it will help you, keep notes of teaching sessions, the goals and plans of the intervention team, and your concerns and worries. No one can be expected to remember everything.

Teaching Methods and Strategies

In many ways, raising your baby with Down syndrome will be the same as raising any other baby. But there will also be many differences. One facet of being the parent of your baby with special needs is the importance of being consciously aware of his development. Babies generally progress automatically from one stage and skill to another. Parents may help them work toward a new goal such as rolling over or reaching out for a toy. But most babies actually direct the efforts and do most of the work. When your baby has Down syndrome, you will have to help direct his development and join him in his "work" to a greater extent.

You may not realize it, but you already know a great deal about your baby. Your knowledge will show when people ask you questions about your baby's likes, dislikes, reactions, and schedules. That knowledge will serve as a useful foundation for everyone's work with your baby.

You will also learn about your baby from your work with professionals. Their help will usually take two forms. First, there will be specific instructions for exercises and activities that will help your baby reach developmental goals. These may require that you set aside a daily period of time, use particular materials, and follow specific teaching methods. For example, you may need to do exercises with your baby to strengthen his abdominal muscles two times a day for several weeks. Or you may need to sit down at a quiet time and use small blocks and a box to help your baby learn to sort shapes. These "lessons" are one part of your baby's early intervention program.

The other major part of your work with your baby requires incorporating developmental goals into everyday activities. Diapering, waking, feeding, bathing, and just sitting with your baby can all be done in ways that promote your child's development. For example, you can hold your baby with his legs together rather than wrapped around your hips (to encourage and reinforce proper leg and hip position), and you can encourage exploration, reaching out, and communication. This added consciousness in your daily parenting is important to your baby's progress. The types of activities and handling techniques can be designed by you and your baby's teachers and therapists. But every baby and every family is different; you will include developmental activities in your child's daily life in ways that fit you, your baby, and your family.

Observing Your Baby

Parents know their children in great detail. As your baby grows and as you learn about development, you will be able to assess your child's developmental strengths and weaknesses, his ways of responding, and his progress. The more you learn about your baby, the better you and your professional partners will be able to develop appropriate ideas for intervention. Observing your baby's everyday activities, movements, and responses is essential for gathering the information you need. In addition to just spotting problems you will wonder at your baby's many accomplishments and strengths.

The following guide for observing your baby's development will help organize the information you may already possess and will give you ideas for additional things to look for. Some questions apply to all levels of development; others are more specific to certain stages. Although these questions can serve as a guide in observing your baby's development, there are, of course, additional questions that you and your baby's teacher will ask.

Responsiveness

- Is he aware of his environment and daily routine?
- Does he seem alert?
- How does he "explore" a new toy? By looking, tasting, holding? For a long time or a short time?
- Does he show any change in response to new places, people, or things?
- Is he generally content? Comfortable? Irritable? Fussy?
- Does he get "keyed up," confused, disorganized, unable to settle down? Can you tell what causes this?
- Does he prefer familiar routines or frequent changes?
- How does he respond to daily activities—bathing, going to sleep, taking naps? Is this predictable or does it vary?
- Does feeding or eating go smoothly? Does it need to be very quiet? How does he respond to new foods—solids, table foods, cup drinking?

Sensory Input

- How does he respond to visual, auditory, tactile, and vestibular (swinging, spinning, and roughhousing) input?
- Does he prefer one type of input to another?
- Does he focus on one kind of input at a time or does he prefer combined activities? For example, does he like toys that have something to watch or something to listen to, or does he like toys that combine both types of input?

Activity and Energy Levels

- What is his energy level throughout the day? Does he seem to be active and alert most of the day or does he tend to have shorter alert periods?
- Is there any consistent pattern? Does he seem to have awake periods in the morning and then again in the late afternoon or does he seem to enjoy playing and interacting most in the early afternoon or evening?
- Are there specific types of activities that he prefers at certain times and not at others?

Preferences

- What types of toys—colorful toys, noisy toys, toys to watch, toys to manipulate, small or large toys—does he prefer?
- Does he have favorite people? Do they seem to have a certain manner of approaching or interacting with him (quiet, high energy, or dramatic)?
- How does he prefer to be held?
- How does he play, move, socialize, and interact with children, adults, and objects?
- Does he prefer structured play or independent play? Structured play is usually started and controlled by an adult, and your baby participates with the adult. Independent play is initiated by your child and directed by him.

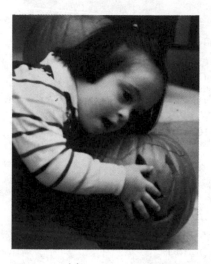

Learning

- Does he seem to do best when activities are short in duration? One structured activity at a time with some independent time in between? Several activities in succession but changed frequently? What activities hold his attention?
- How does he seem to accomplish a new skill? Does he keep trying until he succeeds? Does he try something once and then not for a while? Does he reach one developmental milestone at a time or several at roughly the same time after a long waiting period?
- Does he respond best to familiar activities with new wrinkles added one at a time? Or do new activities seem to motivate him?
- When looking at or listening to new activities, does he seem to stay interested longer if he is in a seat? On the floor? Held in your arms?

Movement

- Does he move about freely and easily or does he prefer to get into a position and stay there for a while?
- How does he position his body during rest and activity?
- What is his preferred resting position—back, side-lying, sitting?
- How does he position his shoulders, arms, hips, knees, legs, feet, and head during movement, rest, and activity?
- Does he move his legs and arms together or reciprocally (one side and then the other)? When?
- Does he use one side of his body more readily than the other?
- Does he reach for and grasp objects easily? Does he work at it repeatedly until he is able to get it?

- How does he hold objects? Does he transfer the object from hand to hand? Hold it in both hands together?
- Does he use his whole hand or just his fingers?
- What does the rest of his body do when he is trying to play with a toy? Does he move freely or stay in a fixed position?

Communication

- Is he generally quiet or does he make noise most of the time?
- Does he make many sounds or mostly repeat the same sounds?
- Does he change from one sound to another although mostly repeating one sound at a time? For example, does your baby say "ba ba *da* ba ba" rather than just repeating "ba?"
- Does he seem to be quiet at certain times and "noisy" at others?
- Do certain activities, movements, or toys (such as mirrors, dolls, and musical toys) motivate "talking?"
- Does he seem to understand very familiar words or names?
- Does he look at you and seem to "talk" to you although he is not saying words? Can you understand his nonverbal communication like pointing, reaching, changing facial expressions?
- Does he have different noises for happy, as opposed to complaining, times?

Not all of the questions above may pertain to your baby right now. These are sample questions, but they will give you an idea of what to begin looking for in getting to know the individual developmental "style" of your baby. This may seem overwhelming, but much of it will become natural and routine. You will be able to see more clearly what activities do and don't work for your baby, how many changes really do occur, and where help is needed. Observe and interact with him; your baby will teach you a great deal about himself. But remember, there are no "right" answers to these questions, they are just for guiding you in observing your child, not in measuring his abilities. Do not use the questions as a developmental checklist. Many perfectly "normal" babies do not perform every skill on any developmental checklist. They don't all score 100 percent or even average. *Every* child—with and without Down syndrome—has his own strengths and weaknesses. The goal is the same—strive to maximize his strengths and minimize his weaknesses.

Teaching Strategies

Because every baby with Down syndrome is unique, no book can prescribe a precise "curriculum" or teaching program for all children. Based on your own observations, on careful developmental evaluations, and on discussions with the professionals involved, you will develop your own comprehensive program.

In working with your child in any program there are many general strategies that can make your work more effective:

- Be as *consistent* as possible. For example, if you tell your baby "no" when he touches the television, it is important that you always tell him "no" when he does this. If you say "no" sometimes and not other times, your baby will be confused about what is expected of him. Consistency is difficult for everyone to achieve and sustain. Be kind to yourself; if you miss an opportunity, just try to get back to your goal. Being consistent in your goals for yourself and for your baby will help foster learning.

- Set *well-defined expectations.* You may want to help your baby put objects into containers. In doing this, your expectation may be that your baby will put three balls into a container on three consecutive days. This will help you be consistent and will make things predictable and measurable. It will also allow you to see when your goals have been accomplished, what your baby has achieved, and when to move to the next step. Ask your child's teacher or therapist to help you set these goals and expectations.

- Divide tasks into *small steps.* If you are helping your baby learn to crawl, a first step may be to place him on his hands and knees and see how long he can stay in that position without your help. The next step could be rocking back and forth in this position, and the third step could be reaching out with one hand while maintaining his hands and knees position. Dividing goals into small steps will again make your work easier by allowing you to identify what part of a task may be difficult for your baby. Again, your child's teacher or therapist can help you with this.

- *Repetition* is a very important part of your baby's learning process. Although you may, at times, feel that it must be boring and that you should change things, watch your baby for cues. Often repetition is precisely what is needed.

- Be *patient and persistent*. Many hard jobs lie ahead. Progress in a particular area may take a long time and can be frustrating for all of you. Don't give up. If you lose patience, remember that it happens to everyone. And just when you are most frustrated, another accomplishment will recharge you.

- A *positive approach* will carry you far. Use of praise and other rewards will motivate your baby and create a positive attitude in both of you. Along with praise, a special book or toy to play with or a favorite song to listen to after a task or part of a task is completed can be used as rewards. Children with Down syndrome—like all children—respond well to praise. Try to praise your baby as soon as possible after he does what you want. But again, no one can do this one hundred percent of the time; it is meant to be a guide—the optimal situation to reach for as much as possible.

- Use *prompts or cues* to help your baby learn, but be sure to give him time to respond. There are a variety of prompts you can give. Physically helping your baby to do an activity may be the most helpful cue you can give. For example, you can hold your child's hands and practice putting a puzzle together. When this kind of help is not necessary, you can try some visual cue or gesture (like pointing) to help your baby begin. A verbal prompt (a reminder of what comes next) can be used with the others from the beginning so that your baby begins to understand what the word or phrase means. For example, while you are physically helping your baby put something into a bucket, also use the verbal prompt "put in." When your baby no longer needs the physical help, he will still understand what "put in" means.

You will undoubtedly find other strategies and teaching methods that work for you and your baby. Be as creative as you can and, most of all, remember that everyone has good times and bad times.

Inclusion

In this chapter, we have spoken about the special services your baby with Down syndrome should receive. These special services are usually provided in an infant program or by private therapists separate from other schools. Parents today, however, are understandably interested in involving their child with special needs in their neighborhood and community schools and classes. This is what is called "inclusion." The principle behind inclusion is that children with disabilities should attend the school or preschool they would attend if they did not have a disability. Support for including children with special needs in regular schools and classes is supported by the federal special education laws which require children with special needs to be educated, to the extent possible, in the "least restrictive environment." This legal concept is discussed in detail in Chapter 8.

Inclusion is a term that came into use in the field of special education recently, although the concept has been around, in different forms, for a long time. Inclusion means being in the main flow of life around you. However valuable and necessary, special education usually means that a child has less contact with his peer group and with his community. Parents and professionals have repeatedly asked how this will affect their children. Frequently the response has been to place children with special needs in regular classrooms.

Inclusion may sound like it applies only to older children but it relates to children of any age and to their families. In addition to providing children with special needs with exposure to regular classes and peer groups, inclusion promotes acceptance from those children and families who do not have the experience of being close to someone with special needs. Being involved with children with special needs and learning to accept them is a valuable social lesson for people of all ages.

Major controversial social questions and much emotion surround the issue of inclusion. It may play a part in your baby's education now or may come to play a part in the future. For now, however, your baby's needs take precedence over the debate about inclusion. For example, your baby may need a very quiet environment with a very small group of children or may need a 1–to–1 student-teacher ratio in order to learn. In this instance, it may be preferable to postpone inclusion in favor of special services.

Inclusion can be either formal or informal. In its informal sense, it means including your baby with Down syndrome in your normal activities, vacations, family visits, neighborhood playgroups, and other typical interactions with neighbors and friends. It means having your baby exposed to the experiences that naturally come with being part of a family.

In its formal sense, inclusion becomes a serious consideration between the ages of two to three years. This is a time when socialization and group experiences become important. It is also a time when you may be looking for a special program with small groups of children with special needs.

Because every child is different, the decision to have your child involved in inclusion is also an individual one. You must assess your child's individual needs and strengths to decide if he would benefit from it. How would he benefit from being part of a neighborhood toddler class? What kind of balance might be achieved to serve all of you best? What kind of special services would be best for him? These are some of the questions to be asked.

It is certainly possible to combine services. Many parents do. If your child is sociable, enjoys watching and being around other children, if he likes small groups and responds well to quite a bit of stimulation, you might want to think about a typical toddler group for at least part of each week. Being in the company of children without special needs can often benefit a young child with Down syndrome in many areas of development. For example, it can be very helpful for language development for your child to be with children who are speaking and communicating in ways he is not. This can provide him with good models and may motivate him to use his language. The same is true of play skills. In a typical class, your child will have opportunities to observe and participate in many varied play experiences.

In inclusion, your child might be placed with children at a similar developmental level. This generally means your child would be placed with children younger than he is chronologically, but with children who share his favorite activities and abilities. Sometimes the models of behavior and communication in a typical toddler class can help your child. He may imitate what he sees other children doing, resulting in a great deal of learning. This of course depends on your child, his needs, your feelings, and the specific program at the community preschool— a lot of considerations to juggle. Ask your early intervention team to work with you: they can help you identify your child's needs and determine what mix of special and typical school experiences would be best.

There are many ways to integrate a child with Down syndrome. Often parents can combine a part-time toddler program in the community with a part-time special early intervention program. For example, three mornings a week your child could be in a special program and two afternoons he could go to a neighborhood toddler class. Or individual physical and speech therapy sessions one to two times a week can complement a typical toddler class. Remember though, the combination of services has to meet your child's needs.

Inclusion can have its drawbacks. This is particularly the case if it precludes getting other special services that your child needs. For example, if your child is learning new things only very slowly and is not speaking or communicating, it may be better for him to be in a smaller, more focused classroom for now. Another drawback of inclusion can result if the neighborhood toddler program cannot or will not use some special teaching techniques for your child, leading to a loss of skills, slower progress, or frustration. It may be that gains in social skills—one of the primary benefits of inclusion—mean that other specific skill areas do not progress as quickly. Your child's progress in all areas of development needs to be monitored and addressed by early intervention specialists if necessary.

Not all private preschools will accept a child with Down syndrome. Unfortunately, some nursery school teachers still refuse to take on children with special needs. Professionals and parents of babies with Down syndrome may know where to direct you to find an accepting program, or you may need to do the searching yourself. Another consideration is that a small neighborhood playgroup might be a good informal alternative to an established preschool program.

If you find a preschool program that will accept your child, it may not be prepared to meet all of your child's special needs and should not necessarily be expected to do so. However, good communication between your child's early intervention team and your child's toddler teachers can be invaluable. Ask your child's teachers if they might talk and exchange ideas. Perhaps each set of teachers can visit the other school (and meet with outside therapists) to learn about how best to intervene with your child. Sharing ideas about how to best help a child with special needs can be very rewarding for all concerned and can give your child the balanced program he needs. You can also carry information and ideas from one program to another. Whatever will work best in your unique situation is the right thing to do.

Conclusion

Early infant education is a complex, dynamic field. As the parent of a baby with Down syndrome, you will learn much about it very quickly. The Reading List at the end of this book contains books on teaching your child and includes several good activity books for parents and children. In addition, the Resource Guide can steer you in the direction of people, agencies, and organizations that can help you get your child started in a program of early intervention. This book has repeatedly pointed out that parents must be responsible for helping their child with Down syndrome reach his full potential. In early intervention, you are indeed your child's primary teacher and evaluator. The work involved in aiding good development is substantial, but getting to know the many facets of your baby and assisting him in reaching toward his potential can be an enriching and rewarding experience as well.

Parent Statements

The parent is always ultimately the case manager.

The whole idea of development and teaching my baby was intimidating in the beginning. I had this picture that I was going to have to work with her ten or twelve hours a day. I thought, "Oh, I just can't." I remember at first trying to do that, but I couldn't keep up with it. Finally I got to the point where I could relax a bit and just enjoy her. And she's probably better off now.

It's a good thing to set aside specific work times if you can. But the best approach to teaching is an incidental approach anyway. Whatever comes up in the routine of the day can be made into a learning experience.

I find myself now in the position of being very protective of new parents I talk to. I let them know they still need to be who they are and go for four days if they feel like going for four days without doing a thing. If that's the way they need to react to their child, that's the way it is. You just can't let the special child be the individual around whom you rotate. You just can't give that much energy.

~ ~ ~ ~ ~ ~ ~

I've always felt that Laurie is a low-tone child. I see her as low tone both mentally and physically. To get her to learn well, you have to hype her up. Music is one of the ways we do it. We use music with a purpose—following directions, sequencing activities, learning concepts. Get her excited and she learns better.

~ ~ ~ ~ ~ ~ ~

Our little girl is in a center-based program. She started at six weeks old. When it first began, she went three times a week; now she goes twice. They have physical therapists, speech therapists, special education teachers, and occupational therapists. She has speech therapy with a group of four kids once a week, and has an individual appointment another day. She gets all the other different teachers randomly. I go to all the sessions with her. It's not hard fitting it all in. I like it because I get out of the house. And she loves it; she loves seeing other children and she loves the toys.

~ ~ ~ ~ ~ ~ ~

Hope's therapists tend to make really vague suggestions, such as "Encourage her to keep trying when something is difficult for her." I've found we get the most useful advice if we ask for specific solutions to specific problems. For example, for the longest time Hope wouldn't hold her own bottle. We asked all the therapists what to do, and one gave us a suggestion that worked—using a bottle straw to help her understand that this was something she could do.

~ ~ ~ ~ ~ ~ ~

The people in the early intervention program pushed us to use Total Communication—signs plus speech—from the start. I wasn't crazy about the idea, as I thought it might delay the development of speech. The first time Hope used the signs for "eat" and "more," though, I was hooked. It made me look at her in a new light—as a little person who knew her own needs and could make them known very capably.

~ ᴗ ~ ᴗ ~ ᴗ ~ ᴗ ~

Learning signs hasn't interfered with our daughter's speech development at all. Often she learns to say the word very shortly after she's learned to use the sign. She learned to sign "bear," and then started saying "beh"; to sign "apple," and then say "a-pull."

~ ᴗ ~ ᴗ ~ ᴗ ~ ᴗ ~

Often I've wished I had someone I could go to for advice on my "normal" child. I always felt it was a great deal to have someone to turn to when I couldn't figure out how to approach a problem—and my special-needs child wasn't the only one to present me with problems!

~ ᴗ ~ ᴗ ~ ᴗ ~ ᴗ ~

I have heard there are a lot of parents who wish they could send their other children to the program, just because it's so good. I visited the classroom and it was cheerful and bright and the teachers seemed genuinely interested; they seemed like they were having a great time.

~ ᴗ ~ ᴗ ~ ᴗ ~ ᴗ ~

The teachers in our program were good. I would go to them really frustrated and feeling unable to set aside an hour to do the things they wanted me to do. But the case manager said, "Look, there are ways that you can incorporate these things into your daily routine—when you're changing her, dressing her, when you're bathing her, and feeding her." When I tried to do that, usually it went a whole lot better. I've pretty much given up trying to do therapy-type work with her at home because she's totally turned off to it now. But if we just play—just start fooling around—then she can learn a lot of things. You have to fake her out. We got these wonderful toys—puzzles, pegboards, and blocks—and all she does is ignore them. I guess she figured out that they were educational.

Some of Hope's therapists have preconceived ideas about what little kids with Down syndrome are like. Even though each child theoretically has his own IFSP, the therapists do the exact same activities with every child with Down syndrome. For example, my daughter crawled very well on her hands and knees at ten months, and there was this other kid in the program who couldn't budge an inch on his own. And yet, the PT kept doing the same exercises with both of them on the therapy ball.

To keep the goals on my daughter's IFSP current, therapists periodically haul out different checklists of skills and behaviors and ask me if she can do certain things. Often when she can't do something, it's because she hasn't had much chance to practice a particular skill. For example, she can't identify x number of clothing items by pointing because I hardly ever say things to her like "OK, let's put your *shirt* on now. Can you hand me your *shirt?* Isn't this a pretty *shirt?*"

It frustrates me that Hope will hardly ever demonstrate what she can really do when someone is assessing her skills. The therapist will try to get her to do something, and she'll just sit there like a lump. So, I'll say, "But she does this all the time when we're alone." Then the therapist will say, "Well, that may be, but let's work on it some more so she can do it more consistently." I guess it's more important that she be able to do something than that she show off, but I hate to waste time on goals she's already accomplished.

❀ ❀ ❀ ❀ ❀ ❀

Fortunately, we have lots of family around to give him his therapy and that's made it a lot easier on us. But even so, we do feel under pressure a little. You know, you feel like if you're free and the kid is sitting there, you should do some exercises with him. There was a time when we pressured him too much and he started refused to do anything and was throwing all his toys around.

❀ ❀ ❀ ❀ ❀ ❀

When we first understood that he had to have intensive therapy, we really got overenthusiastic. We used to make him do exercises until he cried. And we realized that it was just too much; that we were pushing him too hard. He would reject therapy if we made it so painful for him, so we just stopped to reconsider. Now we try to make it fun for him and that's been much more effective. You get little gems of time when you feel you're effective and over time it adds up.

❀ ❀ ❀ ❀ ❀ ❀

She tries really hard on some things. On other things she couldn't care less. She reached a point where she got really turned off about doing certain things—things she didn't like.

❀ ❀ ❀ ❀ ❀ ❀

These children are called "retarded," but they sure can find ingenious ways to avoid having to sit and learn. The old saying that "he may be retarded, but he's not stupid" is really true.

❀ ❀ ❀ ❀ ❀ ❀

We've had a hard time just leaving him to enjoy his quiet time by himself. I feel I should be holding him, stimulating him, dangling a rattle in front of him. It's like we have a higher standard of care because he has Down syndrome.

∼ᴗ∼ᴗ∼∼ᴗ∼ᴗ∼

With the educators you have to trust your feelings and perceptions because you know your child best. We had one therapist who was very good, but whose voice was very shrill, and our son would get upset. It was interfering with his lesson even though the things she was doing were good. So we changed therapists, and found one who was more compatible.

∼ᴗ∼ᴗ∼∼ᴗ∼ᴗ∼

I feel very strongly that if you have a special-needs child you need to explore every option, even if it's an option that doesn't appeal to you at first. I checked out every program, and I talked to many therapists. My husband and I sat together and made lists of the advantages and disadvantages of each thing.

∼ᴗ∼ᴗ∼∼ᴗ∼ᴗ∼

Parents shouldn't have any mental barriers in their own minds about what their child can do because you really can't tell. We were constantly finding that Chris could do things that we had no idea he could do. If we hadn't had therapists and people who knew where to look, we just wouldn't have known. The most striking example was when we first had the speech therapist. He was about nine months old. We had no conception that he could understand words. She got him a ball and a telephone and some of his toys, and she asked him, "Where's the ball?" and he pointed to the ball. She said, "Where's the telephone?" and he pointed to the telephone. We were just so amazed and felt very bad that we didn't know he could do that. Kids can really do a lot more than parents imagine.

∼ᴗ∼ᴗ∼∼ᴗ∼ᴗ∼

Every parent should be linked up with a genetic department somewhere, even if they have to travel once a year sixty miles. I think that with our child a physical therapist was vital in the first year. After the first year, a speech therapist was vital, and once she turned three, an OT was vital. A special education teacher can provide parents with a lot of important information that will carry through for the rest of your child's life—especially in terms of teaching you to be your child's advocate.

We have really felt that the work has paid off. The program has been terrific. It was important because we learned too. They really taught me how to help her and I think that was invaluable, just because I didn't know that much about how to play with babies. I just knew the bare minimum. They taught me a lot about how to play but at the same time teach her. I've learned so much. I can't believe how much I've learned.

You have to figure out what's the most important thing to strive for at each development stage like you do in every child's life and give that input regardless of what a thousand professionals are telling you. You are the case manager and have to figure out what is most important, and let the rest roll off your back, which isn't an easy thing to do.

The teachers at my son's nursery school were very interested in working with him and learning about his special needs. They were especially excited over his accomplishments, maybe because he worked harder than the other kids to achieve things. They also felt more protective, perhaps, toward him than the other children.

Eight

❧❧❧❧❧❧❧

Legal Rights and Hurdles

James E. Kaplan and Ralph J. Moore, Jr.*

Introduction

As the parent of a child with Down syndrome, it is important to understand the laws that apply to you and your child.
There are laws that guarantee your child's rights to attend
school and to live and work in the community. Other laws will
provide your child financial and medical assistance, if she qualifies. Still other laws govern your long-term planning for your
child's future.

It is extremely worthwhile for you to understand how these
laws and principles work. If you know what your child is entitled to, this understanding can help to ensure that your child receives the education, training, and special services she needs to
reach her potential. You will also be able to recognize illegal discrimination and assert your child's legal rights if necessary. Finally, if you understand how laws sometimes create problems

---

* Ralph J. Moore, Jr., and James E. Kaplan are both active in the area of the
legal rights of children with disabilities. They are the co-authors of the
"Legal Rights and Hurdles" chapters in Woodbine House's parents' guides
to children with mental retardation, epilepsy, autism, and cerebral palsy.
Mr. Moore, a partner in the law firm of Shea & Gardner in Washington,
D.C., is the author of *Handbook on Estate Planning for Families of
Developmentally Disabled Persons in Maryland, the District of Columbia, and
Virginia* (Md. DD Council, 3rd edition, 1989). Mr. Kaplan is a principal in
the law firm of Kaplan & Cloutier in Portland, Maine.

for families of children with disabilities, you can avoid unwitting mistakes in planning for your child's future.

There are no federal laws that deal exclusively with Down syndrome. Rather, the rights of children with Down syndrome are found in the laws and regulations for children and adults with disabilities generally. In other words, the same laws that protect all persons with disabilities also protect your child. This chapter will familiarize you with these federal laws to enable you to exercise her rights effectively and fully to protect your child.

It would be impossible to discuss here the law of every state or locality. Instead, this chapter reviews some of the most important legal concepts you need to know. For information about the particular laws in your area, contact the national office of The Arc (formerly the Association for Retarded Citizens) or your local or state affiliate of The Arc. You should also consult

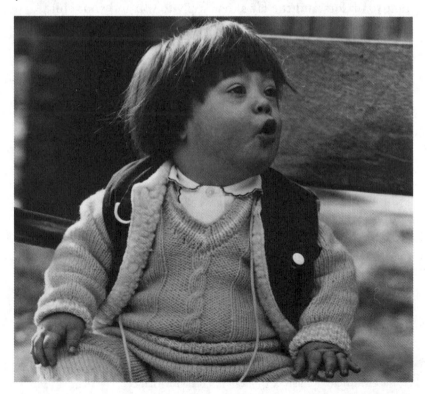

with a lawyer familiar with disability law when you have questions or need specific advice.

Your Child's Right to an Education

Until the middle of this century, children with disabilities were usually excluded from public schools. They were sent away to residential "schools," "homes," and institutions, or their parents banded together to provide private part-time programs. In the 1960s, federal, state, and local governments began to provide educational opportunities to children with disabilities; these opportunities have expanded and improved to this day.

Perhaps nothing has done more to improve educational opportunities for children with Down syndrome as the Individuals with Disabilities Education Act ("IDEA"). This law, originally enacted in 1975, used to be called The Education for All Handicapped Children Act of 1975, but was better known as Public Law 94–142. Along with some recent amendments, the IDEA has vastly improved educational opportunities for almost all children with disabilities. Administered by the U.S. Department of Education and by each state, the law works on a carrot-and-stick basis.

Under the IDEA, the federal government provides funds for the education of children with disabilities to each state that has a special education program that meets federal standards. To qualify for the federal funds, a state must demonstrate, through a detailed plan submitted for federal approval, a policy assuring all children with disabilities a "free appropriate public education." In other words, states accepting federal funds under the IDEA must provide both approved educational services and a variety of procedural rights to children with disabilities and their parents. The lure of federal funds has been attractive enough to induce all states to create special education plans for children with disabilities, including children with Down syndrome.

The IDEA, however, has its limits. The law only establishes the *minimum* requirements in special education programs for states desiring to receive federal funds. In other words, the law *does not* require states to adopt an ideal educational program for your child with Down syndrome or a program that you feel is "the best." Because states have leeway under the IDEA, there are differences from state to state in the programs or services available. For example, the student-teacher ratio in some states is higher than in others and the quality and quantity of teaching materials also can vary widely.

States *can* create special education programs that are better than those required by the IDEA, and some have. Indeed, some state laws impose a higher standard than the federal law requires. Check with the placement or intake officer of the special education department of your local school district to find out exactly what classes, programs, and services are available to your child. Parents, organizations, and advocacy groups continually push states and local school districts to exceed the federal requirements and provide the highest quality special education as early as possible. In addition, these same groups continually urge the federal government to raise the requirements for states under the IDEA. These groups need your support, and you need theirs.

What the IDEA Provides

Since the IDEA was passed in 1975, it has been amended several times. Today the IDEA consists of a large volume of laws and regulations. The Resource Guide at the end of this book tells you how you can obtain copies of these laws and regulations from the U.S. Senate, House of Representatives, or Department of Education. The summary below highlights the provisions most important for you and your child.

Coverage. The IDEA is intended to make special education available to all children with disabilities, including children with mental retardation, hearing impairments, learning disabilities, speech or language impairments, and multiple disabilities. Mental retardation includes any cognitive impairment that "adversely affects...educational performance." In most cases, a diagnosis of Down syndrome is enough to establish that the IDEA applies to your child. Regardless of how your child's intellectual

impairments are labeled, she
qualifies for services if her condition hinders learning.

**"Free Appropriate Pub-
lic Education."** At the heart
of the IDEA is the requirement that children with disabilities receive a "free
appropriate public education."
Children with Down syndrome
are entitled to receive an education at public expense that
takes into account their special learning needs and abili-

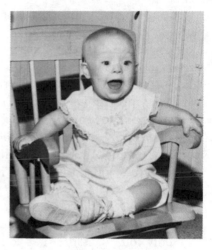

ties. This section examines more precisely what each of the elements of "free appropriate public education" means.

"Free" means that every part of your child's special education program must be provided at public expense, regardless of
your ability to pay. This requirement is often satisfied by placement of your child in a public school, but the school district
must pay the cost of all the necessary services your child will receive there. If no suitable public program is available, the school
district must place your child in a private program and pay the
full cost. Remember, the IDEA does not provide for tuition payment for educational services *not* specifically approved for your
child by the school district or other governing agency (unless, as
explained later in this chapter, the decision of your school district is overturned). As a result, if you place your child in a program the school district does not approve for your child, you risk
having to bear the full cost of tuition.

It may be difficult for parents to accept that the "appropriate" education mandated by the IDEA does not guarantee
either the best possible education that money can buy or even
an educational opportunity equal to that given to children without disabilities. The law more modestly requires only that children with disabilities have access to specialized educational
services individually designed to benefit the child. Interpreting
the IDEA, the United States Supreme Court has stated that a

"free appropriate public education" need not enable a child with disabilities to maximize her potential or to develop self-sufficiency. Instead, a school district can meet the law's requirements in a wide variety of ways. For example, a school district likely would not be required to provide an individual teacher for each student with Down syndrome or provide every child with Down syndrome year-round education even though doing so would maximize that child's educational opportunity. The nature and extent of services provided, however, typically depend on the nature and extent of the need. The law in this area is constantly evolving. Check with your local office of The Arc for information about the current state of the law regarding what is considered an "appropriate" educational program.

Only you can assure that your child receives the most appropriate placement and services. Under the IDEA, parents and educators are required to work together to design an individualized education program (IEP) for each child. If you feel that a school district is not making the best placement for your child, you must demonstrate to school officials not only that your preferred placement is appropriate, but that the placement approved by the school district is not. The goal is to reach an agreement on the appropriate placement. If agreement cannot be reached, there are procedures for resolving disputes. These procedures are discussed later in the chapter.

"Special Education and Related Services." Under the IDEA, an appropriate education consists of "special education and related services." "Special education" means instruction specifically designed to meet the unique needs of the child with disabilities, including as necessary classroom instruction, physical education, home instruction, or instruction in private schools, hospitals, or institutions. Special education teachers, therapists, and other professionals—all provided by the school district at public expense—are responsible for delivering these educational services. "Related services" are defined as transportation and other developmental, corrective, and supportive services necessary to enable the child to benefit from special education.

Related services are often a critical part of a special education program. Services provided by a trained speech or language therapist, occupational therapist, physical therapist, psychologist, social worker, school nurse, aide, or other qualified person may be required under the IDEA as related services. Some services, however, are specifically excluded. Most important among these exclusions are medical services ordinarily provided by a physician or hospital. For example, immunizations cannot be provided as related services under the IDEA.

"Least Restrictive Environment." The IDEA requires that children with disabilities must "to the maximum extent appropriate" be educated in the *least restrictive environment*. The least restrictive environment is the educational setting that permits your child to have the most contact possible at school with children who do *not* have disabilities. Under the IDEA, there is therefore a strong preference to integrate children with disabilities, including children with Down syndrome, in the schools and classes they would attend if they did not have a disability. The IDEA is specifically intended at least in part to end the historical practice of isolating children with disabilities either in separate schools or out-of-the-way classrooms and is intended to open the doors of your neighborhood school to your child with Down syndrome.

Some school officials might assume that all children with Down syndrome should be educated in a separate special setting. Most children with Down syndrome, however, can receive their instruction with typical peers, so long as proper in-classroom supports and therapy are provided. In some localities, all children with disabilities are educated in regular classrooms at all times.

Many children with Down syndrome receive most or all of their instruction and services in regular classes with nondisabled classmates, going to a separate classroom only to receive special services (such as speech therapy) that cannot be provided in the regular classroom. Other children may require more instruction and services in special classes, but nevertheless join the rest of the school for many activities, such as physical education and music, and assemblies and lunch.

The IDEA also recognizes that regular classrooms may not be suitable for all educational and related services required for some children. In these cases, the federal regulations allow for placement in separate classes, separate public schools, private schools, or even residential settings if the school district can demonstrate that this placement is required to meet the child's individual *educational* needs. When placement within the community's regular public schools is determined to be not appropriate, the law still requires that she be placed in the least restrictive educational environment suitable to her individual needs, which can include some participation in regular school classroom programs and activities.

Neither your child's Down syndrome itself nor her developmental delay is a sufficient basis for a school district to refuse to provide opportunities for your child to learn with her typical peers. Some of the most important learning in school comes from a student's peers.

When Coverage Begins under the IDEA. The IDEA requires all states to begin providing special education services from the age of three. In addition, in 1986 Congress amended the IDEA to include grants to states that create an approved program for early intervention services to infants with disabilities from birth through age two. This amendment is sometimes referred to as "Part H" of the IDEA, and allows states to take several years to develop a program for providing early intervention services.

Some form of early intervention services under this program is now available in each state. But there is wide variation in what services are provided, how and where those services are provided, and which agency provides them. You should check with your local school district, the state education agency, or local office of The Arc about the availability of early intervention services which can include speech/language, physical, or occupational therapy to help infants and toddlers with Down syndrome to maximize their early development. Chapter 7 discusses the types of early intervention services your child may receive. You may be charged, however, for some of the early intervention

services your child receives.
The law seeks to have insurance companies and Medicaid
cover some of the costs.

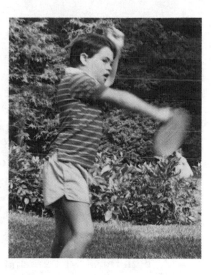

Under the IDEA, special
education services must continue until children reach at
least age eighteen. If a state offers education to all students
until age twenty-one, it must
do the same for students who
receive special education services.

Length of Services. Currently under the IDEA, states
must provide more than the traditional 180–day school year
when the needs of a child indicate that year-round instruction is
a necessary part of a "free appropriate public education." In
most states, the decision to offer summer instruction depends
on whether your child will "regress," or lose a substantial
amount of the progress made during the school year without
summer services. If so, these services must be provided at public expense. Because some children with Down syndrome can regress without year-round services, their parents should not
hesitate to request year-round instruction.

Identification and Evaluation. Because the IDEA applies
only to children with disabilities, your child with Down syndrome must be evaluated before she is eligible for special education. The law requires the states to develop testing and
evaluation procedures designed to identify and evaluate the
needs and abilities of each child before she is placed into a special education program. The evaluation procedure is required to
take into account your input.

For parents of a child with Down syndrome, identification is
somewhat simpler. School districts almost uniformly recognize
that children with Down syndrome need special education. A
medical diagnosis of Down syndrome should therefore be sufficient. Your challenge will not be convincing a school district

that your child is special, but rather obtaining needed services as early as possible. Doctors, organizations, and—most importantly—other parents can be extremely helpful at these initial stages.

"Individualized Education Program." The IDEA recognizes that each child with a disability is unique. As a result, the law requires that your child's special education program be tailored to her individual needs. Based on your child's evaluation, a program specifically designed to address her developmental problems must be devised. This is called an "individualized education program" or, more commonly, an "IEP."

The IEP is a written report that describes:

1. your child's present level of development;

2. both the short-term and annual goals of the special education program;

3. the specific educational services that your child will receive;

4. the date services will start and their expected duration;

5. standards for determining whether the goals of the educational program are being met; and

6. the extent to which your child will participate in regular educational programs.

Under federal regulations, educational placements must be based on the IEP, not vice versa. That is, the services your child receives, and the setting in which she receives them, should be determined by your child's individual needs, not by the availability of existing programs. "One size fits all" is not permitted by the IDEA.

A child's IEP is usually developed during a series of meetings among the parents, teachers, and representatives of the school district. Even your child may be present. School districts are required to establish committees to make these placement and program decisions. These committees are sometimes referred to as Child Study Teams or Administrative Placement Committees.

Writing an IEP is ideally a cooperative effort, with parents, teachers, and school officials conferring on what goals are appropriate and how best to achieve them. Preliminary drafts of the IEP are reviewed and revised in an attempt to develop a mutually acceptable educational program.

The importance of your role in this process cannot be overemphasized. You cannot always depend on teachers or school officials to recognize your child's unique needs. To obtain the full range of services, you may need to demonstrate that withholding certain services would result in an education that would *not* be "appropriate." For example, if you believe that a program using augmentative communication methods is best for your child, you must demonstrate that failing to provide these services would not be appropriate for your child's specific needs. If you want an academic-oriented program for your child, you must demonstrate that a program that emphasizes only vocational or functional skills is not appropriate given your child's skills, abilities, and needs.

IEPs should be very detailed. You and your child's teachers should set specific goals for every area of development, and specify how those goals will be reached. Although the thought of specific planning may seem intimidating at first, a detailed IEP enables you to closely monitor the education your child receives and to make sure she is actually receiving the services prescribed. In addition, the law requires that IEPs be reviewed and revised at least once a year (or more often if necessary) to ensure that your child's educational program continues to meet her changing needs.

Because your child has special needs, her IEP must be written with care to meet those needs. Unless you request specific services, they may be overlooked. You should make sure school officials recognize the unique needs of your child—the needs that make her different from children with other disabilities, and even from other children with Down syndrome.

How can you prepare for the IEP process? First, explore available educational programs, including public, private, federal, state, county, and municipal programs. Observe the classes at the school your child would attend if she did not have Down syndrome to see for yourself what different programs and placements have to offer. Local school districts and local organizations such as The Arc can provide you with information about programs in your community. Second, collect a complete set of developmental evaluations to share with school officials—obtain your own if you doubt the accuracy of the school district's evaluation. Third, give thought to appropriate short-term and long-term goals for your child. Finally, decide for yourself what placement program and services are best for your child, and request them. If you want your child educated in her neighborhood school, request the services necessary to support her in that setting. If no program offers everything your child needs, you should request that an existing program be modified to best meet your child's needs. For example, if your child would benefit educationally from learning sign language, but no programs currently offer such instruction, request the service and suggest how the school district can meet your child's specific needs with existing programs.

To support placement in a particular type of program, you should collect "evidence" about your child's special needs. Then support your position that a particular type of placement is appropriate by presenting letters from physicians, psychologists, therapists (speech/language, physical, or occupational), teachers, developmental experts, or other professionals, as the case may be. This evidence may help persuade a school district that the requested placement or services are the appropriate choices for your child. A few other suggestions to assist you in the process are:

1. Do not attend IEP meetings alone—bring a spouse, advocate, physician, teacher, lawyer, or whomever you would like for support;

2. Keep close track of what everyone—school district officials, psychologists, therapists, teachers, and doctors—involved in your child's case says and does;

3. *Get everything in writing;* and

4. Be assertive and speak your mind. Children with unique developmental challenges need parents to be assertive

and persuasive advocates during the IEP process. This does not mean that school officials are always adversaries, but does mean you are your child's most important advocate; you know her best.

"Individualized Family Service Plan." Parents of children from birth through age two use a plan that is different from the IEP used for older children. States receiving grants to provide early intervention services must draft an "individualized family service plan" (IFSP). This plan is similar to the IEP with an early intervention focus. Unlike an IEP, which focuses primarily on the needs of the child, an IFSP emphasizes services for the family. In other words, the law recognizes that families with young children with special needs often have special needs themselves. Consequently, IFSPs do not simply specify what services are provided for the child with Down syndrome. They also describe services that will be provided to: 1) help parents learn how to use daily activities to teach their child with Down syndrome; and 2) help siblings learn to cope with having a brother or sister with Down syndrome. The procedures and strategies for developing a useful IFSP are the same as described above for the IEP. IFSPs are reviewed every six months.

Resolution of Disputes under the IDEA

The IDEA establishes a variety of effective safeguards to protect your rights and the rights of your child. For instance, written notice is always required before any change can be made in your child's identification, evaluation, or educational placement. In addition, you are entitled to review all of your child's educational records at any time. Further, your school district is prohibited from deceiving you and from making decisions without consulting or notifying you first.

Despite these safeguards, conflicts between parents and school officials can arise. When they do, it is usually best to resolve disputes over your child's educational or early intervention program *during* the IEP or IFSP process, before hard positions have been formed. Although the IDEA establishes dispute resolution procedures that are designed to be fair to parents, it is easier and far less costly to avoid disputes by reaching agreement if possible during the IEP or ISFP process or by informal discussions with appropriate officials. Accordingly, you should first try to accomplish your objectives by open and clear communication and by persuasion. If a dispute arises that simply cannot be resolved through discussion, further steps may be taken under the IDEA and other laws to resolve that dispute.

First, the IDEA allows you to file a formal complaint with your local school district about *any matter* "relating to the identification, evaluation, or educational placement of the child, or the provision of free appropriate public education to such child." This means that you can make a written complaint about virtually any problem with any part of your child's educational or early intervention program. This is a very broad right of appeal, one that parents have successfully used in the past to correct problems in their children's education programs.

The process of challenging a school district's decisions about your child's education can be started simply by sending a letter of complaint. This letter, which should explain the nature of the dispute and your desired outcome, typically is sent to the special education office of the school district. You have the absolute right to file a complaint—you need not ask the school district for permission to do this. For information about starting appeals, you can contact your school district, your local office of The Arc, local advocacy groups, or other parents.

The first step in the appeal process is usually an "impartial due process hearing" before a hearing examiner. This hearing, usually held on the local level, is your first opportunity to explain your complaint to an impartial person, who is required to listen to both sides and then to render a decision. At the hearing, you are entitled to be represented by a lawyer or lay advocate; you can present evidence; and you can examine, cross-examine, and compel witnesses to attend. Your child has a right to be present at the hearing as well. After the hearing, you have a right to receive a written record of the hearing and the hearing examiner's findings and conclusions.

Just as with the IEP and IFSP processes, you must present facts at a due process hearing that show that the school district's decisions about your child's educational program are wrong. To overturn the school district's decision, you must show that the disputed placement or program does not provide your child with the "free appropriate public education" in "the least restrictive environment" that is required by the IDEA. Evidence in the form of letters, testimony, and expert evaluations is usually essential to a successful challenge.

Parents or school districts may appeal the decision of a hearing examiner. The appeal usually goes to the state's educational agency or to a neutral panel. The state agency is required to

---

IMPORTANT NOTICE TO OUR READERS:

Congress is currently considering proposals to amend the IDEA to significantly reduce this law's mandates to the states to provide a free appropriate public education to children with disabilities in the least restrictive environment. If the proposed legislation becomes law, the information in this chapter may be superseded. As your child's primary advocate, you may want to contact your congressperson and senators to express your concern about this important law.

---

make an independent decision upon a review of the record of the due process hearing and of any additional evidence presented. The state agency then issues a decision.

The right to appeal does not stop there. Parents or school officials can appeal beyond the state level by bringing a lawsuit under the IDEA and other laws in a state or federal court. In this legal action, the court must determine whether there is a preponderance of the evidence (that is, whether it is more likely than not) that the school district's placement is proper for that child. The court must give weight to the expertise of the school officials responsible for providing your child's education, al-

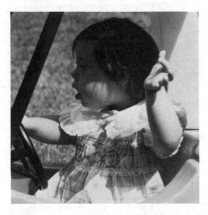

though you can and should also present your own expert evidence.

During all administrative and judicial proceedings, the IDEA requires that your child remain in her current educational placement, unless you and your school district or the state education agency agree to a move. If you place your child in a different program without an agreement, you risk having to bear the full cost of that program. If the school district eventually is found to have erred, it may be required to reimburse you for the expenses of the changed placement. Accordingly, you should never change programs without carefully considering the potential cost of that decision.

Attorneys' fees are another expense to consider. Parents who ultimately win their dispute with a school district may recover attorneys' fees at the court's discretion. Even if you prevail at the local or state level (without bringing a lawsuit), you likely are entitled to recover attorneys' fees. A word of caution: A court can limit or refuse attorneys' fees if you reject an offer of settlement from the school district, and then do not obtain a better outcome. In addition, if you sue the school district under Section 504 of the Rehabilitation Act of 1973 (discussed below), you may be entitled to attorneys' fees under that law.

As with any legal dispute, each phase—complaint, hearings, appeals, and court cases—can be expensive, time-consuming, and emotionally draining. As mentioned earlier, it is wise to try to resolve problems without filing a formal complaint or bringing suit. When informal means fail to resolve a problem, formal channels should be pursued. Your child's best interests must come first. The IDEA grants important rights that you should not be bashful about asserting vigorously.

The IDEA is a powerful tool in the hands of parents. It can be used to provide unparalleled educational opportunities to your child with Down syndrome. The Reading List at the end of this book includes several good guidebooks to the IDEA and the special education system. The more you know about this vital law, the more you will be able to help your child realize her fullest potential.

Programs and Services When Your Child Is an Adult

Many children with Down syndrome grow to live independently or semi-independently as adults. To achieve community living and employment skills, your child may need some special services. These services include employment, job-training, and residential or community-living programs. Regrettably, these services are often unavailable because very few federal laws require states to offer programs for adults with disabilities. Those programs that exist typically are underfunded and have long waiting lists. As a result, many parents must provide the necessary support and supervision on their own for as long as possible. Thousands of children receive education and training that equip them to live independently and productively, only to be sent home when they finish schooling with nowhere to go and nothing to do.

Now is the time to attempt to change this sad reality. The unemployment rate for people with Down syndrome is appallingly high, especially for young adults. As waiting lists for training programs grow, your child may be deprived of needed services, and, consequently, of her independence. Programs sponsored by charities and private foundations are limited and most families do not have the resources to pay the full cost of providing employment and residential opportunities. The only other remedy is public funding. Just as parents banded together in the 1970s to demand enactment of the IDEA, parents must band together now to persuade local, state, and federal officials to take the steps necessary to allow adults with disabilities to live in dignity. Parents of *children* with disabilities should not leave this job to parents of *adults* with disabilities; children become adults all too soon.

Vocational Training Programs

One educational program supported by federal funding is available to most adults with Down syndrome. Operating somewhat like the IDEA, federal law makes funds available to states to support vocational training and rehabilitation programs for qualified people with disabilities. As with the IDEA, states that desire federal funds for this program must submit plans for approval. Unlike the IDEA, however, these laws do not contain enforceable rights and procedures.

Adults must fulfill two requirements to qualify for job-training services: 1) they must have a physical or mental disability that constitutes a "substantial handicap to employment"; and 2) they must be expected to benefit from vocational services. In the past, some people with Down syndrome were denied vocational training services because it was believed that they would never be able to meet the law's second requirement of being expected to perform full-time or part-time employment. Recent amendments to the law, however, require that services and training be provided to people even if what they achieve is "supported employment," which means employment in a setting with services such as a job coach or special training that allows an individual to work productively.

The state Departments of Vocational Rehabilitation, sometimes called "DVR" or "Voc Rehab," are charged with administering these laws. Adults who apply for Voc Rehab services are evaluated, and an "Individualized Written Rehabilitation Plan" (IWRP) or an "Individualized Habilitation Plan" (IHP), similar to an IEP, is developed. The IHP sets forth the services needed to enable a person with a disability to work productively.

You should contact your state vocational rehabilitation department or your local office of The Arc for specific information on services available to your child. Despite shrinking federal and state budgets, some states and communities offer their own programs, such as group homes, supported employment programs, and life-skills classes. Other parents and organizations likely will have information about these local programs.

Developmentally Disabled Assistance and Bill of Rights Act

Under a federal law called the Developmentally Disabled Assistance and Bill of Rights Act, states can receive grants for a variety of programs. Important among them is a protection and advocacy (P&A) system. A P&A system advocates for the civil and legal rights of people with developmental disabilities. P&A offices have been leaders in representing institutionalized people with Down syndrome seeking to improve their living conditions or to be placed in the community. In addition, P&A offices may be able to represent persons who cannot afford a lawyer for an IDEA due process hearing or a discrimination suit. Because people with Down syndrome may not be able to protect or enforce their own rights, state P&A systems offer necessary protection. Consult the Resource Guide at the back of this book for the location of your state's P&A office.

Anti-Discrimination Laws

In a perfect world, no one would be denied opportunities or otherwise discriminated against solely on the basis of disability, race, sex, or any other factor beyond her control. Unfortunately, our world remains imperfect, and the federal government has enacted several laws to ensure that children, adolescents, and adults with disabilities be given the right to live and work in the community to the fullest extent possible. This section reviews the highlights of the landmark Americans with Disabilities Act and the Rehabilitation Act of 1973, both of which prohibit discrimination against your child with Down syndrome and all people with disabilities.

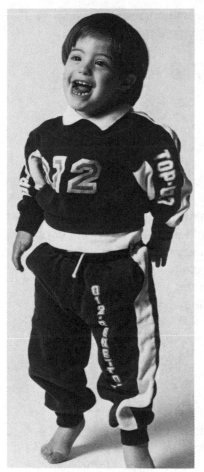

The Americans with Disabilities Act of 1990

The Americans with Disabilities Act (ADA) prohibits discrimination against people with disabilities, including children and adults with Down syndrome. The law is based on and operates in the same way as other well-known federal laws that outlaw racial, religious, age, and sex discrimination. The ADA applies to most private employers, public and private services, public accommodations, businesses, and telecommunications.

Employment. The ADA states that no employer shall discriminate against a qualified individual with a disability "in regard to job application procedures, the hiring or discharge of employees, employee compensation, advancement, job training, and other terms, conditions, and privileges of employment." In other words, private employers cannot discriminate against employees or prospective employees who have a disability. The law defines "qualified individual with a disability" as a person with a disability who, with or without reasonable accommodation, can perform the essential functions of a job. "Reasonable accommodation" means that employers must make an effort to remove obstacles from the job, the terms and conditions of employment, or the workplace that would prevent an otherwise qualified person from working because she has a disability. Accommodations can include job restructuring, schedule shuffling, modified training and policies, and access to readers or interpreters. Failing to make reasonable accommodations in these respects is a violation of this law.

The law does not *require* employers to hire people with disabilities or to make accommodations if an "undue hardship" will result for the employer. Rather, employers may not refuse to employ qualified people with disabilities solely because of the existence of the disability. For example, if a person with Down syndrome applies for a job as a file clerk in an office, the employer may not refuse to hire her if she was as qualified as or *more* qualified than other applicants to perform the job's duties and the employer's refusal was based on the applicant's Down syndrome. The employer is not required to hire qualified people with Down syndrome, but cannot refuse to hire a person who otherwise can perform the job because of her disability. The employer may not either inquire whether the applicant has a disability or fail to make some reasonable accommodation to enable a person with Down Syndrome to work productively. The employment section of the ADA applies only to companies that employ fifteen or more persons.

The ADA specifies procedures for people with disabilities who believe they have been the victim of employment discrimination. A person must file a complaint with the federal Equal Employment Opportunity Commission (EEOC), the agency responsible for resolving employment discrimination complaints. If the agency does not satisfactorily resolve the dispute, a lawsuit may be brought in court to prohibit further discrimination and to require affirmative action. The ADA allows an award of attorneys' fees to a person with a disability who wins a lawsuit. The local Arc may be able to provide basic information about how to challenge discriminatory employment practices, but a lawyer likely will be required.

Public Accommodations. One of the most stunning and potentially far-reaching provisions of the ADA is the prohibition of discrimination in public accommodations. Mirroring the approach of the civil rights laws of the 1960s, the ADA bans discrimination against people with disabilities virtually *everywhere,* including hotels, inns, and motels; restaurants and bars; theaters, stadiums, concert halls, auditoriums, convention centers, and lecture halls; bakeries, grocery stores, gas stations, clothing stores, pharmacies, and other retail businesses; doctor or lawyer offices; airport and bus terminals; museums, libraries, galleries, parks, and zoos; nursery, elementary, secondary, undergraduate, and postgraduate schools; day care centers; homeless shelters; senior citizen centers; gymnasiums; spas; and bowling alleys. Virtually any place open to the public must also be open to people with disabilities, unless access is not physically or financially feasible. No longer can businesses exclude people with disabilities just because they are different. The excuse that people with disabilities are "not good for business" is now unlawful thanks to the ADA.

For example, a theater, restaurant, or museum cannot exclude people with Down syndrome from their facilities, cannot restrict their use to certain times or places, and cannot offer them only separate programs, unless to do otherwise would impose unreasonable cost on these facilities. The end result is that the new law simply it does not merely prohibit active discrimination, but rather imposes duties to open our society to all people with disabilities.

Like other civil rights laws, the ADA also requires integration. The law bans the insidious practice of "separate but equal" programs or facilities that offer separate services to people with disabilities, rather than access to programs offered to everyone else. The law prohibits the exclusion of people with disabilities on the grounds that there is a "special" program available for them. For example, a recreation league (public or private) could not uniformly exclude people with disabilities on the ground that a comparable separate league is offered.

People who are the victims of discrimination can file a lawsuit to prohibit further discrimination. And if the U.S. Department of Justice brings a lawsuit to halt a pattern and practice of discrimination, monetary damages and civil penalties may be imposed. Again, the local office of The Arc and state P&A office will be able to provide information and assist in a discrimination complaint.

The ADA provides extraordinary freedom and opportunity to people with Down syndrome. By prohibiting discrimination and requiring reasonable accommodation, the ADA stands as

> **IMPORTANT NOTICE TO OUR READERS:**
>
> Congress is currently considering legislation to amend or revoke the ADA. If this proposed legislation becomes law, the information in this section may be superseded. As your child's primary advocate, you should contact your congressional representatives to express your concern about this important law.

the Bill of Rights for people with all disabilities, including Down syndrome.

The Rehabilitation Act of 1973

Before the ADA was enacted, discrimination on the basis of disability was prohibited only in certain areas. Section 504 of the Rehabilitation Act of 1973 continues to prohibit discrimination against qualified people with disabilities in *federally funded programs.* The law provides that "No otherwise qualified individual with handicaps in the United States . . . shall, solely by reason of his handicap, be excluded from the participation in, be denied the benefits of, or be subjected to discrimination under any program or activity receiving federal financial assistance. . . ."

An "individual with handicaps" is any person who has a physical or mental impairment that substantially limits one or more of that person's "major life activities," which consist of "caring for one's self, performing manual tasks, walking, seeing, hearing, speaking, breathing, learning, and working." The United States Supreme Court has determined that an "otherwise qualified" handicapped individual is one who is "able to meet all of a program's requirements in spite of his handicap."

Programs or activities that receive federal funds are required to make reasonable accommodation to permit the participation of qualified people with disabilities. This can include programs like day care centers and schools and jobs in programs receiving federal funds.

Section 504 has been used to enforce the right of children with disabilities to be integrated in their school district, to challenge placement decisions, and to assert the right to special education services for children who do not qualify for services under IDEA. Even if a child functions at a level that disqualifies her from services under IDEA, her right to services may be enforceable under Section 504. In addition, Section 504 permits the recovery of reasonable attorneys' fees. This may be important for parents of very high functioning children with Down syndrome. Every local education agency is required to have a Section 504 Coordinator to answer questions. As with other legal issues, you should consult a qualified attorney to explore claims under Section 504.

Health Insurance

Often the mere fact of a child's Down syndrome can cause serious problems for families in finding and maintaining health insurance that covers the child. Unfortunately, most insurance companies do not offer health or life insurance at a fair price, or sometimes at any price, to children or adults with Down syndrome. This practice results from the belief that these children and adults are likely to submit more insurance claims than others. Until they become adults, children who are covered from birth by their parents' insurance face fewer problems, but this depends on the particular terms of the insurance.

About half the states have laws against handicap-based discrimination that prohibit insurance companies from denying coverage based on a disability like Down syndrome. The drawback to all of these laws, however, is that insurance companies are allowed to deny coverage based on "sound actuarial principles" or "reasonable anticipated experience." Insurers rely on these large loopholes to deny coverage. In short, the laws often are ineffective in protecting families from insurance discrimination. Even the ADA does not prohibit these same "sound actuary" practices that frequently result in denied coverage.

A few states have begun to lessen the health insurance burdens on families with children with disabilities. These states have passed insurance reform laws that prohibit exclusion of children with disabilities from coverage. Other states offer "shared risk" insurance plans, under which insurance coverage is offered to people who could not obtain coverage otherwise. The added cost is shared among all insurance companies (including HMOs) in the state. To be eligible, a person must show that she has been recently rejected for coverage or offered a policy with limited coverage. The cost of this insurance is usually higher and the benefits may be limited, but it is usually better than no health insurance at all. Some state laws also cover people who have received premium increases of 50 percent or more. In addition, Medicare and Medicaid may be available to help with medical costs. Check with your state insurance commission or your local office of The Arc for information about health insurance programs in your area.

Planning for Your Child's Future: Estate Planning

Although some children with Down syndrome grow into independent adults, others are never able to manage completely on their own. This section is written for parents whose children may need publicly funded services or assistance, or help in managing their funds when they are adults.

The possibility that your child may be dependent all of her life can be overwhelming. To properly plan for your child's future, you need information in areas you may never have considered before. In most families, parents remain primarily responsible for ensuring their child's well-being. Consequently, questions that deeply trouble parents include: "What will happen to my child when I die? Where and with whom will she live? How will her financial needs be met? Who will provide the services she may need?"

Some parents of children with Down syndrome delay dealing with these issues, coping instead with the immediate demands of the present. Others begin to address the future when their child is quite young. They add to their insurance, begin to set aside funds for their child, and share with family and friends their concerns about their child's future needs. Whatever the course, parents of children with Down syndrome need to understand in advance of any action some serious problems that affect planning for the future. Failure to avoid these pitfalls can have dire future consequences for your child and for other family members.

There are three important issues that families of children with Down syndrome need to consider in planning for the future. These are:

1. the potential for cost-of-care liability;
2. the complex rules governing government benefits; and
3. the child's ability to handle her own affairs as an adult.

Of course, there are many other matters that may be different for parents of children with Down syndrome. For example, life insurance needs may be affected, and the important choice of trustees and guardians is more difficult. But these types of concerns face most parents in one form or another. Cost-of-care liability, government benefits, and the inability to manage one's own affairs as an adult, however, present concerns that are unique to parents of children with disabilities.

Cost-of-Care Liability

Fewer and fewer people with Down syndrome reside in state-run facilities, but some still do, and many receive residential services paid for in part by the state. When a state provides residential services to a person with disabilities, it often requires her to pay for them if she has the funds to do so. Called "cost-of-care liability," this requirement allows states to tap the funds of the person with disabilities herself to pay for the services the state provides. States can reach funds owned outright by a person with disabilities and even funds set aside in some trusts. Some impose liability for services like day care and vocational training, in addition to residential care. Some states even impose liability on parents for the care of an adult with disabilities. This is an area parents need to look into early and carefully.

You should understand clearly that payments required to be made to satisfy cost-of-care liability do *not* benefit your child. Ordinarily they add nothing to the care and services a person with disabilities receives. Instead, the money is added to the general funds of the state to pay for roads, schools, public officials' salaries, and so on.

It is natural for you to want to pass your material resources on to your children by will or gift. In some cases, however, the unfortunate effect of leaving your child with Down syndrome a portion of your estate may be the same as naming the state in your will—something most people would not do voluntarily, any more than they would voluntarily pay more taxes than the law requires. Similarly, setting aside funds in your child's name, in a support trust, or in a Uniform Transfers to Minors Act (UTMA) account may be the same as giving money to the state—money that could better be used to meet the future needs of your child.

What, then, can you do? The answer depends on your circumstances and the law of your state. Here are three basic strategies parents use:

First, strange as it may seem, in some cases the best solution may be to disinherit your child with Down syndrome, leaving funds instead to siblings in the hope that they will use these funds for their sibling's benefit, even though they will be under no *legal* obligation to do so. The absence of a legal obligation is crucial. It protects the funds from cost-of-care claims. The state will simply have no basis for claiming that the person with disabilities owns the funds. This strategy, however, runs the risk that the funds will not be used for your child with Down syndrome if the siblings: 1) choose not to use them that way; 2) suffer financial reversals or domestic problems of their own, exposing the funds to creditors or spouses; or 3) die without making arrangements to safeguard the funds.

A preferable method in many cases, in states where the law is favorable, is to leave funds intended for the benefit of your

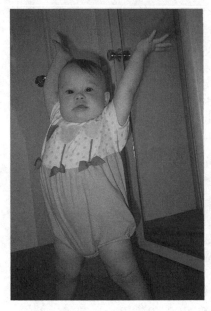

child with Down syndrome in what is called a "discretionary" special-needs trust. This kind of trust is created to supplement, rather than replace, money the state may spend on your child's care and support. The trustee of this kind of trust (the person in charge of the trust assets) has the power to use or not use the trust funds for any particular purpose as long as it benefits the beneficiary—the child with Down syndrome. In many states, these discretionary trusts are not subject to cost-of-care claims because the trust does not impose any *legal* obligation on the trustee to spend funds for care and support. In contrast, "support" trusts *require* the trustee to use the funds for the care and support of the child and can be subjected to state cost-of-care claims. Discretionary trusts can be created under your will or during your lifetime; as with all legal documents, the trust documents must be carefully written. In some states, to protect the trust against cost-of-care claims, it is necessary to add provisions stating clearly that the trust is to be used to supplement rather than replace publicly funded services and benefits.

A third method to avoid cost-of-care claims is to create a trust, either under your will or during your lifetime, that describes the kind of allowable expenditures to be made for your child with Down syndrome in a way that excludes care in state-funded programs. Like discretionary trusts, these trusts—sometimes called "luxury" trusts—are intended to supplement, rather than take the place of, state benefits. The state cannot reach these funds because the trust forbids spending any funds on care in state institutions or programs.

In using these estate planning techniques, you should consult a qualified attorney who is experienced in estate planning for parents of children with disabilities. Because each state's laws differ and because each family has unique circumstances, individualized estate planning is essential.

Government Benefits

A wide variety of federal, state, and local programs offer financial assistance for people with disabilities. Each of these programs provides different services and each has its own complicated eligibility requirements. What parents and grandparents do now to provide financially for their child with Down syndrome can have important effects on that child's eligibility for government assistance in the future. In addition, the complex rules governing some programs—such as Medicaid—can have far-reaching effects on your child's life.

SSI and SSDI

There are two basic federally funded programs that can provide additional income to people with Down syndrome who cannot earn enough to support themselves. The two programs are "Supplemental Security Income" (SSI) and "Social Security Disability Insurance" (SSDI). SSI pays monthly checks to senior citizens and to children and adults with serious disabilities who lack other income and resources. SSDI pays a monthly check to adults disabled from work who are either covered by Social Security based on past earnings, or whose disability began before age eighteen and who are the children of deceased or retired persons who earned Social Security coverage. Both SSI and SSDI are designed to provide a monthly income to people with disabilities who meet the programs' qualifications. Both programs are administered by the Social Security Administration. There are additional programs that may provide financial assistance to people with disabilities, including children of deceased federal employees, military personnel, and railroad employees.

Qualifying for SSI. If your child qualifies for SSI, she will receive monthly payments from the Social Security Administration (SSA) to "supplement" your family's income. As of 1995, the *maximum* individual payment provided through SSI was $458 per month for an individual and $687 for an eligible married couple. In order to receive SSI benefits, an applicant must establish that she is "disabled." To qualify as "disabled," the applicant's condition must be so disabling that she cannot engage in "substantial gainful activity." This means that she cannot perform any job, whether or not a suitable job can be found. The Social Security Administration regulations prescribe a set of tests for making this determination. The test of severity is somewhat different for children and adults.

The SSA has changed its regulations to allow more children to qualify as disabled. This is because the U.S. Supreme Court held in 1990 that the rules for determining which disabilities qualify children for SSI benefits were too restrictive and discriminatory. However, Congress is currently considering legislation that would reverse the Court's ruling, and reduce sharply the number of children who will be able to qualify for SSI.

SSI's eligibility requirements do not end with the test of severity. Eligibility for SSI is also based on financial need. An applicant is ineligible to receive SSI benefits if her assets (including property owned in her own name and income she is entitled to receive under a trust) exceed a certain level. Currently, that level is $2,000 for an individual and $3,000 for a couple. In addition, for children under eighteen years of age who live at home, the resources of the parents are also considered. In general, children with disabilities are eligible only if their parents' income is quite restricted.

Many people with Down syndrome work. In fact, for most parents, finding a job for their child with Down syndrome is a goal they strive hard to achieve. It is an unfortunate irony that earning a salary can affect eligibility for SSI and SSDI. Under the rules governing SSI benefits, earning income can reduce your child's benefits or disqualify her altogether. This is because, as presently administered, SSI is intended to provide income to people whose disabilities prevent them from working.

This rule is unfair to people with Down syndrome who are able to perform work because it can force a choice between work in the community at reduced pay and needed SSI benefits. People receiving SSI, however, *can*, under a statutory work incentive program, earn up to a certain amount (now $1,001 per month) and still keep *some* SSI benefits; the benefits will be reduced by the amount of excess income earned. In addition, under the PASS program (Plans for Achieving Self-Support), a recipient can receive income or assets in her own name, provided the funds will be used to make it possible for the SSI recipient to work in the future or to establish a business or occupation that will enable her to become gainfully employed.

Unless she participates in the PASS program, however, your child will be ineligible for SSI if she has assets in her own name greater than a prescribed level (now $2,000). The assets of parents are deemed to be assets of their children under age eighteen in determining eligibility, so most children with disabilities first become eligible when they reach age eighteen. It is vital to properly plan your child's financial future to avoid jeopardizing her right to receive SSI benefits. You should check periodically with the Social Security Administration to determine the current rules that apply to your child.

Qualifying for SSDI. People with disabilities may also qualify for SSDI—disability benefits under the Social Security program. The test for disability is the same as it is for SSI. People do not have to be poor to qualify for SSDI, unlike SSI, however; there are no financial eligibility requirements based on resources or unearned income. To be eligible, an applicant must qualify on the basis of her own work record for Social Security purposes, or she must be unmarried, have a disability that began before age eighteen, and be the child of a parent covered by Social Security who has retired or died.

As with SSI, your child's employment can cause serious problems. The work incentive program under SSI does not apply to people on SSDI, who lose eligibility if they earn more than a certain amount per month (now $500), because they are deemed not to be disabled. Again, this rule places an unfair burden on recipients of SSDI by forcing them to make a choice between work and financial security. Recently, however, a new program under SSDI allows recipients to work for one year on a trial basis without losing eligibility to determine their ability to work.

Medicare

Medicare is a federal health insurance program that helps pay for the medical expenses of people who qualify. People who are eligible for SSDI benefits, either on their own account or on a parent's account, will also be eligible for Medicare, starting at any age, after a waiting period. These persons will automatically receive Part A (hospital) coverage, and they can elect Part B (medical) coverage, for which they will pay a premium. If a person can also qualify for Medicaid, discussed below, Medicaid may pay the Medicare Part B premium. In some cases, children or adults with disabilities who would not otherwise be eligible for Medicare may qualify if a third party—parents, relatives, charities, or even state and local governments—pay into Medicare. Called "third party buy-in," this works very much like purchasing private health insurance. Check with your local Social Security Administration office for details.

Medicaid

Medicaid is also important to many people with Down syndrome. It pays for medical care for people who do not have private health insurance or Medicare and lack sufficient income to pay for medical care. It also pays for residential services for many people with disabilities. It is funded partly by the states and partly by the federal government, and is administered by the states. In most states, if your child meets the eligibility criteria for SSI, she will qualify for Medicaid when she reaches age eighteen. Because eligibility is based on financial need, however, placing assets in the name of your child with Down syndrome can disqualify her.

It is important for you to become familiar with the complex rules governing SSI, SSDI, Medicare, and Medicaid. Always feel free to contact your local Social Security Administration office, or call the national toll-free number (800/772–1213). And as discussed below, it is even more important to avoid a mistake that could disqualify your child from receiving needed benefits.

Competence to Manage Financial Affairs

Even if your child with Down syndrome may never need state-funded residential care or government benefits, she may need to have her financial affairs managed for her. Care must be exercised in deciding how to make assets available for your child. There are a wide variety of trusts that can allow someone else to control the ways in which money is spent after you die. Of course, the choice of the best arrangements depends on many different circumstances, such as your child's capacity to manage assets, her relationship with her siblings, your financial situation, and the availability of an appropriate trustee or financial manager. As an adult, your child will want to be consulted regarding decisions that affect her; you should arrange for that. Each family is different. A knowledgeable lawyer can review the various alternatives and help you choose the one best suited to your family.

Need for Guardians

Parents frequently ask whether they should nominate themselves or others as guardians once their child with Down syndrome becomes an adult. The appointment of a guardian costs money and may result in the curtailment of your child's civil rights—the right to marry, to have a checking account, to vote, and so on. Therefore, a guardian should be appointed only if and when needed. If one is not needed during your lifetime, it usually is sufficient to nominate guardians in your will.

A guardian will be needed if your child inherits or acquires property that she lacks the capacity to manage. Also, a guardian may be required if a medical provider refuses to serve your child without authorization by a guardian. Occasionally it is necessary to appoint a guardian to gain access to important legal, medical, or educational records. Unless there is a specific need that can be solved by the appointment of a guardian, however, a guardianship should not be established simply because your child has Down syndrome.

Life Insurance

Parents of children with Down syndrome should review their life insurance coverage. The most important use of life insurance is to meet financial needs that arise if the insured person dies. Many people who support dependents with their wages or salaries are underinsured. This problem is aggravated if hard-earned dollars are wasted on insurance that does not provide the amount or kind of protection that could and should be purchased. It is therefore essential for any person with dependents to understand basic facts about insurance.

The first question to consider is: Who should be insured? Life insurance deals with the *financial* risks of death. The principal financial risk of death in most families is that the death of the wage earner or earners will deprive dependents of support. Consequently, life insurance coverage should be considered primarily for the parent or parents on whose earning power the children depend, rather than on the lives of children or dependents.

The second question is whether your insurance is adequate to meet the financial needs that will arise if you die. A reputable insurance agent can help you determine whether your coverage is adequate. Consumer guides to insurance listed in the Reading List of this book can also help you calculate the amount of insurance you need.

The next question is: What kind of insurance policy should you buy? Insurance policies are of two basic types: term insurance, which provides "pure" insurance without any build-up of cash value or reserves, and other types (called "whole life," "universal life," and "variable life"), which, in addition to providing insurance, include a savings or investment factor. The latter kinds of policies are really a combined package of insurance and investment. The different types of insurance are described in more detail in the consumer guides to insurance listed in the Reading List of this book.

People with children who do not have disabilities try to assure that their children's educations will be paid for it they die before their children finish their educations. Many people use life insurance to deal with this risk. When their children are grown and educated, this insurance need disappears. Term insurance is a relatively inexpensive way to deal with risks of this kind.

On the other hand, people with Down syndrome are likely to need supplemental assistance throughout their lives. That need will not disappear completely during their parents' lifetimes. If the parents plan on using life insurance to help meet this need when they die, they must recognize, in deciding what kind of insurance to buy, that term insurance premiums rise sharply as they get older. Consequently, they should either consider a savings or investment program to eventually replace the insurance, or consider purchase of whole life or universal life.

Whether you buy term insurance and maintain a separate savings and investment program, or instead buy one of the other kinds of policies that combines them, you should make sure that the insurance part of your program is adequate to meet your family's financial needs if you die. A sound financial plan will meet these needs and will satisfy savings and retirement objectives in a way that does not sacrifice adequate insurance coverage.

Finally, it is essential to coordinate your life insurance with the rest of your estate plan. This is done by designating the beneficiary—choosing who is to receive any insurance proceeds when you die. If you wish any or all of these proceeds to be used for your child's support, you may wish to designate a trustee in your will or in a separate revocable life insurance trust. Upon your death, the trustee will receive the insurance proceeds and use them to benefit your child in accordance with the trust. If you do not have a trustee, your child's inheritance may be subject to the cost-of-care claims, or may interfere with eligibility for government benefits, described earlier.

A Guide to Estate Planning for Parents of Children with Down Syndrome

More than most parents, the parents of a child with Down syndrome need to attend to estate planning. Because of concerns about cost-of-care liability, government benefits, and competency, it is vital that you make plans. Parents need to name the people who will care for their child with Down syndrome when they die. They need to review their insurance to be sure it is adequate to meet their child's special needs. They need to make sure their retirement plans will help meet their child's needs as an adult. They need to inform grandparents of cost-of-care liability, government benefits, and competency problems so that grandparents do not inadvertently waste resources that could otherwise benefit their grandchild's future. Most of all, they need to make a will so that their hopes and plans are realized and the disastrous consequences of dying without a will are avoided.

Proper estate planning differs for each family. Every will must be tailored to individual needs. There are no formula wills, especially for parents of a child with Down syndrome. There are, however, some common mistakes to avoid. Here is a list:

No Will. If parents die without first making wills, state law generally requires that each child in the family share equally in the parents' estate. The result is that your child with Down syndrome will inherit property in her own name. Her inheritance may become subject to cost-of-care claims and could jeopardize eligibility for government benefits. These and other problems can be avoided with a properly drafted will. Do not ever allow your state's laws to determine how your property will be divided upon your deaths. Estate planning can make you feel uneasy, but it is too important to ignore.

A Will Leaving Property Outright to the Child with Down Syndrome. Like having no will at all, having a will that leaves property to a child with Down syndrome in her own name may subject the inheritance to cost-of-care liability and may disqualify her for government benefits. Parents of children with Down syndrome do not just need any will, they need a will that meets their special needs.

A Will Creating a Support Trust for Your Child with Down Syndrome. A will that creates a support trust presents much the same problem as a will that leaves property outright to a child with Down syndrome. The funds in these trusts may be subject to cost-of-care claims and jeopardize government benefits. A will that avoids this problem should be drafted.

Insurance and Retirement Plans Naming a Child with Down Syndrome as a Beneficiary. Many parents own life insurance policies that name a child with Down syndrome as a beneficiary or contingent beneficiary, either alone or in common with siblings. The result is that funds may go outright to your child with Down syndrome, creating cost-of-care liability and government benefits eligibility problems. Parents should designate the funds to pass either to someone else or to go into a properly drawn trust. The same is true of many retirement plan benefits.

Use of Joint Tenancy in Lieu of Wills. Spouses sometimes avoid making wills by placing all their property in joint tenancies with right of survivorship. In joint tenancies, property is owned equally by each spouse; when one spouse dies, the survivor automatically becomes the sole owner. Parents try to use joint tenancies instead of wills, relying on the surviving spouse to properly take care of all estate planning matters. This plan, however, fails completely if both parents die in the same disaster, if the surviving spouse becomes incapacitated, or if the surviving spouse neglects to make a proper will. The result is the same as if neither spouse made any will at all—the child with Down syndrome shares equally in the parents' estates. As explained above, this may expose the assets to cost-of-care liability and give rise to problems with government benefits. Therefore, even when all property is held by spouses in joint tenancy, it is necessary that both spouses make wills.

Establishing UTMA Accounts for Your Child with Down Syndrome. Over and over again well-meaning parents and grandparents open bank accounts for children with disabilities under the Uniform Transfers to Minors Act (UTMA).

When the child reaches age eighteen or twenty-one, the account becomes the property of the child, and may therefore be subject to cost-of-care liability. Perhaps more important, most people with disabilities first become eligible for SSI and Medicaid at age eighteen, but the UTMA funds will have to be spent before financial eligibility for these programs can be established. Parents should *never* set up UTMA accounts for their child with Down syndrome, nor should they open other bank accounts in the child's name.

Failing to Advise Grandparents and Relatives of the Need for Special Arrangements. Just as the parents of a child with Down syndrome need properly drafted wills or trusts, so do grandparents and other relatives who may leave (or give) property to the child. If these people are not aware of the special concerns—cost-of-care liability, government benefits, and competency—their plans may go awry and their generosity may be wasted. Make sure anyone planning gifts to your child with Down syndrome understands what is at stake.

Children and adults with Down syndrome are entitled to lead full and rewarding lives. But many of them cannot do so without continuing financial support from their families. The *only* way to make sure your child has that support whenever she needs it is to plan for tomorrow today. Doing otherwise can rob her of the future she deserves.

Conclusion

Parenthood always brings responsibilities. But extra responsibilities confront parents of a child with Down syndrome. Understanding the pitfalls for the future and planning to avoid them will help you to meet the special responsibilities. In addition, knowing and asserting your child's rights can help guarantee that she will receive the education and government benefits to which she is entitled. Being a good advocate for your child requires more than knowledge. You must also be determined to use that knowledge effectively, and, when necessary, forcefully.

Parent Statements

In getting your child placed in the best program, you have to work your own kid's needs out first. You have to understand your child first of all, and then you have to go in and argue your case. But it's something you can anticipate. You see it coming, and you can start to do some book-learning, and you can get ready.

When we learned that the private therapists were doing an even better job, we just dropped the public program. My feeling was that since we could afford it and this period of time was so crucial, we had to have the best. It was worth it for us. We're spending our time and energy and resources getting him the therapy he needs rather than trying to get the public agency to get them.

Parents need the law explained to them. They've got a club with which they can demand some rights. It helps to find other parents who are slightly ahead of them, and get counsel from them.

By law, early intervention programs are supposed to determine what services each kid in the program needs and then provide them with those services. But what our county's program does is to look at what therapists they have available, and then parcel the therapists' services out among the kids. If they don't have enough speech therapists to meet every kid's needs, then tough luck. First come, first served. I don't know what it would take to force the county to obey the law.

The early years are so important to our son that we work very hard to make sure he gets the best education possible. Our school district has good intentions, but sometimes needs to be shown the way. We're polite, but we are also prepared and very persistent.

～ ～ ～ ～ ～ ～

Under the law [IDEA], it's all based on what is an "appropriate" education for Mike. When the school district says "appropriate" it may mean just "appropriate;" but when I say "appropriate" I mean "best."

～ ～ ～ ～ ～ ～

We have a special trust for Chris that is protected from invasion by the state. But we've done more than that. The best insurance that we have for our child is our family and our relatives. I know my family would take care of Chris as much as they could. We named guardians in our will in the event of our deaths. We sent a letter to the relatives who were named in the will and the trust and that gave us an important sense of security.

～ ～ ～ ～ ～ ～

We've resisted disinheriting Hope, because to us that means admitting that she will never be truly independent as an adult. We just aren't emotionally ready for that step yet.

～ ～ ～ ～ ～ ～

We think a lot about the boys and how they will be settled in about twenty years or so. We'd like to see Josh in a group home. We make our decisions with that in mind. We always make decisions based on the long term. We don't think too much about the day-to-day stuff.

～ ～ ～ ～ ～ ～

With estate planning, you just have to grin and bear it and realize you're in for the long haul. You have to start planning for it now. Parents have the obligation to find out what the facts and circumstances are and get competent advice, and then explain the situation to grandparents. It's sometimes difficult to raise the issue, but you have to, or there can be unintended consequences.

We want Josh to grow into a person who can function on his own, with a little structure here and there. We want him to help take care of himself. There may come a day when he has to fend for himself. We want him to be able to do that.

We feel strongly that we don't want her sister to feel in any way responsible in the long term. We feel that what happens will happen, but a lot will come from the attitude of how you bring your children up to care about each other.

I know it sounds selfish, but my greatest worry is that within a few years doctors and scientists will find a way to eliminate Down syndrome so our children might be the last generation of people with Down syndrome. If that happens, there might not be good services any longer.

Getting competent advice doesn't necessarily mean going to a high-priced lawyer. It can be as easy as finding whatever advocacy program exists in your community, whether through the Arc or a group who specializes in helping people with Down syndrome. It really helps to find out if they have advocacy programs for parents, and take a course.

Our hope is that he will be able to be a wage earner and tax-payer, and pay back to the community at least part of what they have given him. I think he can accomplish it. I know his schools have been very expensive for the county, but it's all worthwhile.

～◡～◡～◡～◡～

I've read that so far, very few people with mental retardation have been able to use the ADA to their advantage. The main people who have benefitted from it are alcoholics who were having problems getting or keeping jobs and successfully argued that alcoholism is a disability. That makes me mad! Obviously, it pays to know how to play the system—but how many kids with disabilities and their parents do?

～◡～◡～◡～◡～

When I was growing up, the only time I ever saw kids with disabilities was at Christmas. Once a year, my high school honor society would go over to this segregated school called "Sunny Acres" and give a party for the kids. Frankly, I hated doing this. The kids at the school were always starved for attention and would swarm all over us. They all wore mismatched clothes and smelled like they should have had their diapers changed hours ago. I just felt like they belonged in their world, and I belonged in mine, and that was the best for everyone concerned. Today, thanks to laws like the IDEA and ADA, our kids *should* grow up with much more enlightened and tolerant nondisabled peers. Hopefully, at least some of the "normal" kids they come in contact with will honestly want to be their friends.

GLOSSARY

Abstractions—Concepts, symbols, and principles that cannot be experienced directly, such as time and space.

Actuarial—The process of using statistics to calculate risks and life expectancy for insurance providers.

ADA—See *Americans with Disabilities Act.*

Adaptive behavior—The ability to adjust to new environments, tasks, objects, and people, and to apply new skills to those new situations.

Adenoids—Pads of lymph tissue located behind the nose and nasal cavity.

Advocacy groups—A wide variety of organizations that work to protect the rights and opportunities of children with disabilities and their parents.

Alpha-A-Crystallin Gene—The gene that controls the amount of protein in the lens of the eye. This gene may be connected to cataracts.

Alpha-feto protein (AFP)—A protein present in the blood of pregnant women. Abnormally low amounts of it may indicate that the fetus has Down syndrome.

Alzheimer's disease—A degenerative disease of the brain that causes the gradual loss of mental ability. May affect older people with Down syndrome.

Amblyopia—Loss of vision caused by a variety of eye problems, including nearsightedness, farsightedness, and crossed eyes. Also called *lazy eye.*

Americans with Disabilities Act (ADA)—The law that prohibits discrimination by employers, government agencies, and *public accommodations* against people with disabilities, including people with Down syndrome.

Amniocentesis—A method to test the cells of a fetus for possible genetic defects. A needle is inserted through the mother's belly and a small amount of *amniotic fluid* is withdrawn. The chromosomes within the cells are then tested.

Amniotic fluid—The liquid that surrounds an embryo in a woman's uterus.

Amyloid Beta Protein Gene—A gene that controls the production of certain proteins in the brain. May be related to *Alzheimer's disease.*

Antibiotics—A group of drugs that kills bacteria that cause illness.

Assessment—An *evaluation* of the strengths, needs, and developmental progress of a child. Assessments are used to help design education services.

Astigmatism—An irregularity in the shape of the eyeball which prevents light waves from focusing properly on the retina. Blurred vision results.

Atlantoaxial instability—Instability in the joints of the upper bones of the *spinal column.*

Atria—The two upper chambers of the heart.

Atrial septal defect (ASD)—A defect—often a small hole—in the wall between the two upper chambers of the heart.

Atrioventricular canal defect (AV Canal)—A defect in the structure of the heart in which the walls of the two upper chambers and the two lower chambers may be deformed.

Attention span—The length of time a child stays on task or is able to pay attention to one thing (attending).

Audiologist—A professional trained to evaluate and measure hearing and hearing impairments. He or she also fits hearing aids.

Auditory—Having to do with sounds; the ability to hear.

Auditory Brainstem Response (ABR)—A test that measures electronically the brain's reception of sound. It is used to measure hearing in infants who cannot give verbal responses to sound. Also called auditory evoked potential, auditory evoked response, and evoked response audiometry.

Babbling—The sound a baby makes when he combines a vowel and consonant and repeats them over and over again (e.g. ba-ba-ba, ga-ga-ga).

Bell curve—A curve on a graph that shows the distribution of characteristics in a population. These curves are used to show the range of human intelligence and developmental skill acquisition, as well as many other characteristics of populations.

Beneficiary—The person designated in a trust or insurance policy to receive any payments that become due.

Bilateral—Relating to or affecting both sides of a child's body; of importance in developing skills. For example, banging a drum with two hands.

Blood Pressure—The pressure the flow of blood exerts on the arteries.

Bone Marrow Transplant (BMT)—A treatment for leukemia in which healthy bone marrow is transplanted to replace cancerous bone marrow.

Brachycephaly—A condition in which the back of the skull is somewhat flatter than normal.

Bronchitis—Inflammation of the bronchial tubes, the two branches of the windpipe.

Brushfield spots—Light spots on the outer part of the iris of the eyes, often an outward manifestation of Down syndrome.

Cardiac—Having to do with the heart.

Cardiac catheterization—A surgical diagnostic technique in which a *catheter* is passed into the heart so that *blood pressure* and blood flow can be measured and viewed.

Cardiac surgeon—A doctor who specializes in heart surgery.

Cardiologist—A doctor specializing in diagnosing and treating heart conditions.

Case Manager—The person on a child's educational or medical multidisciplinary team who is responsible for coordinating all members of the team.

Cataracts—A disease of the eye that causes the lens to become cloudy or opaque, resulting in partial or total blindness.

Catheter—A flexible tube that is used to provide or remove fluids from the body.

Cause-and-effect—The concept that actions create reactions.

Center-based program—An early intervention program that is provided at a center—a school, health center, or private office.

Chemotherapy—A treatment for leukemia (and other diseases) that uses chemicals to kill cancer cells.

Child-centered service—A type of early intervention program that focuses solely on the child with disabilities.

Chorionic villus sampling (CVS)—A method for testing the *chromosomes* of an embryo at nine to eleven weeks of pregnancy. A small number of fetal cells are removed from the chorion (the outside of the placenta) through a *catheter* inserted through the cervix into the uterus. The cells' *chromosomes* are then tested.

Chromosomes—Microscopic rod-shaped bodies in the nucleus of every cell of the body that contain genetic material.

Clinical geneticist—A doctor who specializes in the study and diagnosis of genetic disorders.

Cognition—The process of perceiving, thinking, reasoning, and analyzing.

Colic—A condition of some young infants in which the baby has abdominal pain.

Communication skills—The ability to use language to receive and express information and emotion.

Congenital—A condition that exists at the time of birth.

Congenital heart defect—A defect of the heart present at birth.

Consequence—The result of an action; an approach to discipline that emphasizes the natural results of a child's action or behavior.

Coordination—Synchronized, balanced, or harmonious muscle movements.

Cost-of-care liability—The right of a state providing care to a person with a disability to charge for the care and to collect from the person's assets.

Cradle cap—A patch of crusty dry skin on the scalp of newborns that flakes off over time. This condition is normal in babies.

Crawling—To use the arms and legs to move the body along the floor with the abdomen on the floor.

Creeping—To use the arms and legs to move the body along the floor with the abdomen off the floor.

Critical region—The part of the number-21 chromosome thought to be responsible for the majority of differences seen in Down syndrome.

Crossed eyes—A condition in which one eye is turned inward while the other eye looks straight ahead. Also known as *esotropia* (when eyes turn inward) or *exotropia* (when eyes turn outward), this condition can cause double vision.

Cruising—Standing and moving on two feet while holding onto a support such as a table.

Cue—*Input* that prompts a child to perform a behavior or activity.

Culture—A medium in which microscopic organisms are grown, such as blood samples used in *karyotypes.*

Cyanosis—A bluish color of skin caused by a lack of oxygen in the blood. This can occur in babies with heart defects.

Cytogeneticist—A doctor who studies *chromosomes.*

Daughter cells—The two cells created during *mitosis* that are exact copies of the parent cell.

Decongestant—A type of medicine that relieves congestion of the nasal passages and allows freer breathing.

Development—The process of growth and learning during which a child acquires skills and abilities.

Developmental milestone—A developmental goal that acts as a measurement of developmental progress over time, such as an infant rolling over between two and four months of age.

Developmental pediatrician—A doctor who specializes in the development of infants and children. Often he or she is part of an educational multidisciplinary team.

Developmental delay—Development that is slower than normal.

Developmental disability—A condition that prevents a person from developing normally.

Dietitian— A professional with a degree in nutrition or dietetics who is registered and may have a state license. This professional offers advice and counselling regarding improving or modifying food intake for optimal nutrition.

Digoxin—A drug used to treat congestive *heart failure* which increases the force of heart contractions.

Discretionary trust—A trust in which the trustee (the person responsible for governing the trust) has the authority to use or not use the trust funds for any purpose, as long as funds are expended only for the beneficiary.

Disinherit—To deprive someone (such as a person with a disability) of an inheritance. Parents of children with disabilities may do this to prevent the state from imposing cost-of-care liability on their child's assets.

Disjunction—The process by which *chromosomes* separate during *meiosis.*

Dispute resolution procedures—The procedures established by the IDEA and regulations for the fair resolution of disputes regarding a child's special education.

Diuretics—Drugs that increase the flow of urine, resulting in a decrease in the amount of fluid in the body. They are often used to help children with heart defects to reduce the heart's load because accumulated fluids tend to stress the heart.

DNA—Deoxyribonucleic acid, the spiral-shaped molecule that carries hereditary traits.

Down syndrome—A common genetic disorder in which a person is born with forty-seven rather than forty-six *chromosomes,* resulting in developmental delays, mental retardation, low muscle tone, and other effects.

Down syndrome clinics—Clinics, often affiliated with universities, that specialize in treating the medical conditions of people with Down syndrome.

Dramatic play—Play involving imagination, role-playing, and games of make-believe. The ability to engage in dramatic play is regarded as a measure of cognitive and social development.

Due process hearing—Part of the procedures established to protect the rights of parents and children with disabilities during disputes under the *IDEA.* These are hearings before an impartial person to resolve disputes related to the identification, evaluation, placement, and services by a child's educational agency.

Duodenal atresia—A narrowing or blockage of the first part of the small intestine.

EAHCA—The Education for All Handicapped Children Act of 1975, also called Public Law 94–142. This landmark law established the right of children with Down syndrome and other disabilities to a *"free appropriate public education."* See *IDEA.*

Ear tubes—Also called *myringotomy,* these small tubes are inserted in the eardrum to allow the fluid to drain from the middle ear and also ventilate the middle ear.

Early development— Development during the first three years of life.

Early intervention—Providing therapies and other specialized services to minimize the effects of conditions such as Down syndrome that can delay *early development.*

Echocardiogram (EKG)—A painless test that uses high-frequency sound waves to create an image of the heart.

The Education For All Handicapped Children Act of 1975 (EAHCA)—The former name of Public Law 94–142, which guarantees a *"free appropriate public education"* to children with disabilities. See *IDEA*.

EEOC—Equal Employment Opportunity Commission. A federal agency that is responsible for resolving employment discrimination complaints under the *Americans with Disabilities Act*. Complaints must first be made to the EEOC before a lawsuit may be brought.

Egg—The female reproductive (sex) cell.

Electrocardiogram (ECG)—A medical instrument that measures the electrical impulses of the heart. These measurements show a cardiologist how a heart is functioning and can reveal heart disease.

Embryo—A baby in the earliest stages of development in the uterus.

Endocardial cushion defect—Defects or deformations in the walls between the chambers of the heart.

ENT Physician—Ear, Nose, and Throat Physician.

Epicanthal folds—Small folds of skin in the inner corners of the eyes. Often present in babies with Down syndrome.

Epilepsy—A neurological condition in which a person has seizures—periods of unconsciousness or convulsions.

Equilibrium—Balance.

Esotropia—See *crossed eyes*.

Estate planning—Formal, written arrangements for handling the possessions and assets of people after they have died.

ETs-2 gene—This gene, found on the number-21 chromosome, is called an *oncogene*. It is involved in cancer or leukemia.

Eustachian tube—A small tube between the middle of the ear and the back of throat that controls air pressure in the ear and drains fluids from the *middle ear*. This tube can become blocked by fluid, resulting in a loss of hearing.

Evaluation—The process of determining the developmental level of a child. Evaluations are used to determine if a child needs educational services, as well as to determine what types of services he needs. The evaluation consists of a series of tests covering all areas of development.

Expressive language—The ability to use gestures, words, and written symbols to communicate.

Extension—The straightening of the muscles and limbs.

Facilitation—A teaching technique of helping a baby or child to perform a task or activity.

Family-centered service—A type of early intervention program that focuses on the child and his or her family as a whole.

FAPE—See *Free Appropriate Public Education.*

Farsightedness—A condition of the eye that causes near objects to be seen blurred and objects in the distance to be seen clearly. Also called *hypermetropia*, this condition can be corrected with glasses.

Fine motor—Involving movements of the small muscles of the body, such as the hands, feet, fingers, and toes.

Flexion—The bending of the muscles and limbs.

Fontanels—The soft spots of the skull; the spaces between the separate bones of the skull.

Free Appropriate Public Education (FAPE)—The basic right to special education established under the *Individuals with Disabilities Education Act.*

Gastrointestinal system—The stomach and intestines that function to digest food.

Generalization—Using a skill learned in one situation in another. Using information about an object or concept to make conclusions about a similar object or concept.

Genes—Contained within the *chromosomes*, genes contain the hereditary material. Each gene controls specific traits.

Genetic Code—The pattern of proteins on human DNA that determines hereditary traits.

Genetics—The study of *genes, chromosomes,* and heredity.

Germ cell—The cell that results when a *sperm* cell (male) combines with an *egg* cell (female).

Grasp—The way a person holds an object.

Gross motor—Involving movements of the large muscles of the body.

Hand-eye coordination—The use of the eyes to guide the hands in movements, such as picking up an object.

Hearing aid—A device that amplifies sounds for people who have a *hearing impairment.*

Hearing impairment—Loss of hearing; a decrease in the ability to hear sounds of different volume and pitch.

Heart defects—*Congenital* abnormalities of the heart.

Heart failure—A condition of the heart in which it is unable to function at the optimal level.

Heart valves—Tissue inside the heart that seals off the chambers during heart contractions to force blood to flow in only one direction.

Hirschsprung's disease—A condition in which there are no nerve cells in the colon (large intestine). It appears during early infancy and causes the colon to distend.

HMO—Health Maintenance Organization.

Home-based program—An *early intervention* program that provides services at home.

Hyperextensive joints—Joints (such as the hips or shoulders) that are unusually flexible.

Hypermetropia—See *farsightedness.*

Hypothyroidism—The decreased production of thyroid hormone by the thyroid gland. This condition is more common in babies with Down syndrome than in other children, but is easily treated.

Hypotonia—Low muscle tone; see *muscle tone.*

IDEA—The Individuals with Disabilities Education Act. This law establishes the right of children with Down syndrome and other disabilities to a *"free appropriate public education."*

Identification—The determination that a baby or child should be evaluated as a possible candidate for special education services.

IEP—See *Individualized Education Program.*

IFSP—See *Individualized Family Service Plan.*

IHP—See *Individualized Habilitation Plan.*

Imitation—The ability to observe the actions of others and to copy them in one's own actions.

Immunization—The process of making a person immune to certain diseases, using injections or other methods.

Imperforate anus—A *congenital* condition in which the anal opening is either absent or obstructed.

Inclusion—The practice of having children with Down syndrome and other disabilities attend the same school and classes they would attend if they did not have a disability.

Individualized Education Program (IEP)—A written report that details the *special education* program to be provided a child aged three and older with a disability. Sometimes referred to as IPP or Individualized Program Plan.

Individualized Family Service Plan (IFSP)—A written report that details the *early intervention* services to be provided to an infant with Down syndrome or other disability.

Individualized Habilitation Plan (IHP)—A written report that sets forth the services needed to enable a person with a disability to learn to work productively.

Individualized Written Rehabilitation Plan (IWRP)—See *Individualized Habilitation Plan.*

Individuals with Disabilities Education Act—See *IDEA.*

Infant—A child under 12 months of age.

Infant educator—A teacher trained to work on helping with the overall development of infants, and specifically with cognitive development.

Infant stimulation—A term that was used in the past to describe *early intervention*.

Input—Information that a child receives through any of the senses such as vision, hearing, touch, or feeling that helps him or her develop new skills or respond to his environment.

Intellectual impairment—A term used to describe or substitute for *mental retardation*.

Intelligence quotient (IQ)—A numerical measure of a child's intelligence or cognitive ability as determined by *standardized tests*.

Interactive play—Children playing with each other.

Interpretive—The session during which parents and teachers review and discuss the results of a child's *evaluation*.

Intestinal malformation—A condition of the intestine, such as a blockage, that prevents the normal function of the gastrointestinal tract.

IWRP—See *Individualized Habilitation Plan*.

Jargon—The usually-unintelligible speech of *infants* and young children that is a stage in the development of full expressive speech.

Joint tenancy—Property that is owned equally by each spouse; when one spouse dies, the survivor automatically becomes the sole owner.

Karyotype—A picture of human *chromosomes* made after culturing of cells from a fetus or person. These can reveal the presence of extra genetic material.

Language—The expression and understanding of human communication.

Large muscles—Muscles such as those in the arms, legs, and abdomen.

Lazy eye—See *amblyopia*.

Least Restrictive Environment (LRE)—The requirement under the *IDEA* that children with disabilities receiving special education must be made a part of a regular school to the fullest extent possible. Included in the law as a way of ending the traditional practice of isolating children with disabilities.

Leukemia—A type of cancer that attacks the red blood cells. This disease is slightly more common among children with Down syndrome.

Local education agency (LEA)—The agency responsible for providing educational services on the local (city, county, school district) level.

Luxury trust—A trust that describes the kind of allowable expenses in a way that excludes the cost of care in state-funded programs in order to avoid *cost-of-care liability*.

Mainstream—A term for the practice of involving children with disabilities in regular school and preschool environments. See *Inclusion*.

Medicaid—A federal program that offers medical assistance to people who are entitled to receive *Supplementary Security Income*.

Medicare—A federal program that provides payments for medical care to people who are receiving Social Security payments.

Meiosis—The process of the development of reproductive (sex) cells (*egg* and *sperm*) during which the number of *chromosomes* is usually reduced by half to 23. Upon conception, the fertilized egg usually has 46 *chromosomes*.

Mental retardation—Below average mental function combined with below average adaptive behavior. Children who have mental retardation learn more slowly than other children, but "mental retardation" itself does not indicate the child's level of cognitive ability. The degree of mental function may not be identifiable until a much later age.

Metatarsus varus—Abnormal toeing in of the foot.

Microcephaly—Head size that is at or below the third percentile on "normal" growth charts.

Middle ear fluid—Fluid that accumulates in the middle ear, behind the eardrum. It interferes with hearing, and can lead to hearing loss if not treated. Technically called *otitis media*.

Midline—The vertical center of the body. Development progresses from the midline (proximal) to the extremities (distal). Some important developmental activities occur at the midline (e.g. bringing hands together at the midline) because they allow for other important developmental gains.

Mitosis—The process of cell division during which a cell produces an exact copy of itself, including a duplicate set of chromosomes.

Mosaicism—A rare type of Down syndrome in which a faulty cell division occurs in one of the first cell divisions after fertilization. The result is that some but not all of the baby's cells contain extra genetic material.

Mottled skin—Spotted or blotchy skin color or skin with variable color.

Muscle tone—The degree of elasticity or tension of muscles when at rest. Can be too low *(hypotonia)* or too high *(hypertonia)*; either condition causes developmental problems, particularly in motor areas. Children with Down syndrome commonly have low muscle tone.

Myopia—See *nearsightedness*.

Myringotomy—A surgical procedure to create a small opening in the eardrum to allow fluid to drain from the *middle ear*. Often, an *ear tube* is placed to maintain the opening.

Nasal bridge—The bony structure at the top of the nose between the eyes. Usually flatter in babies with Down syndrome.

Naso lacrimal duct obstruction—Blocked tear ducts.

Nearsightedness—A condition of the eye that causes objects in the distance to be seen blurred and near objects to be seen clearly. Called *myopia*, this condition can be corrected with glasses.

Neurodevelopmental Treatment (NDT)—An approach to therapy that emphasizes discouraging abnormal patterns of posture and movement and facilitates the greatest possible variety of innate normal basic motor patterns. Used by physical, occupational, and speech therapists.

Nondisjunction—The failure of sex cell (*egg* and *sperm*) *chromosomes* to separate properly during *meiosis*. This can be a cause of *Nondisjunction Trisomy 21*.

Nondisjunction Trisomy 21—The most common type of Down syndrome, caused by the failure of chromosome number 21 to separate during meiosis in the egg (female) or sperm (male).

Nucleotides—The chemical building blocks of *DNA*.

Nutritionist—An individual who provides advice about diet and nutrition.

Obesity—Excessive weight or fat; when a person exceeds their recommended weight by 20 percent.

Object permanence—The cognitive understanding that objects exist even when they are out of sight.

Occupational therapist (OT)—A therapist who specializes in improving the development of fine motor and adaptive skills.

Oncogene—A *gene* that is linked to cancer.

Oral motor—Relating to the use of the muscles in and around the mouth and face. Oral motor skills are important for learning to eat and talk properly.

Orthopedic inserts—Small devices placed in shoes to help stabilize the ankles and feet. Sometimes used to help children with Down syndrome because of low muscle tone and flexible joints. Also called orthotics.

Open heart surgery—Surgery during which the chest and heart are opened to enable surgeons to make repairs to the heart.

Ophthalmologist—A medical doctor who specializes in diagnosing and treating conditions of the eyes.

Otitis Media—See *Middle Ear Fluid*.

Oxygenate—The process of tissue absorbing oxygen delivered by the blood.

Parallel play—Children playing near each other and in the same way, but without interacting.

Parent-professional partnership—The teaming of parents and teachers (or doctors, nurses, or other professionals) to work together to facilitate the development of babies and children with special needs.

Part H of IDEA—The provisions in *IDEA* that make early intervention services available to babies with Down syndrome and other disabilities.

Partial Trisomy 21—A rare condition in which the extra 21st chromosome in the cells of a child with Down syndrome is missing part of its genetic material. Which characteristics of Down syndrome are present depends on which portion of the 21st chromosome is present.

PASS (Plans for Achieving Self-Support)—A *SSI* program in which a SSI recipient can receive income or assets in her own name, provided the funds will be used to make it possible for him or her to work in the future or to establish a business or occupation that will enable him or her to become gainfully employed.

Patching—One treatment for *amblyopia*, in which a child's good eye is covered in order to force the weaker eye to develop.

Patellar instability—Instability of the kneecap.

Pediatric cardiologist—A doctor who specializes in diagnosing and treating heart conditions in children.

Pediatric geneticist—A doctor who studies genes and the effects of genetic conditions in children.

Pediatric ophthalmologist—A doctor who specializes in the care and treatment of the eyes of children.

Periodontal disease—Disease of the gums and bones surrounding the teeth.

Pes planus—Flat feet.

Physical therapist (PT)—A therapist who works with a baby or child to help him overcome physical problems such as low *muscle tone* or weak muscles.

Pincer grasp—The use of the thumb and forefinger to grasp small objects.

Placement—The selection of the educational program for a child who needs *special education* services.

Pneumonia—An inflammation of the lungs resulting from an infection.

Posture—How a person stands or carries him or herself.

Precursors—Behaviors or skills that precede the development of more sophisticated behaviors or skills.

Prompt—*Input* that encourages a child to perform a movement or activity.

Protection & Advocacy (P&A)—A nationwide system providing legal services for families of children with disabilities, including Down syndrome.

Public Accommodation—A place, such as a school, restaurant, or theater, generally open to the public. The *ADA* prohibits discrimination against people with disabilities by public accommodations.

Public Law 94–142—The Education for All Handicapped Children Act of 1975, which provides for a *"free appropriate public education"* for children with disabilities. This law applies to children with Down syndrome. Its name was changed to the *Individuals with Disabilities Education Act (IDEA)*.

Public Law 99–457—The law which established *early intervention* services for infants with disabilities, including infants with Down syndrome. This law is now *Part H* of *IDEA*.

Pulmonary hypertension—High *blood* pressure in the blood vessels in the lungs. This condition can result from *heart defects* that cause excessive amounts of blood to be pumped to the lungs, and can be fatal if not corrected.

Pyloric stenosis—A narrowing of the opening between the stomach and the duodenum, the first part of the small intestine.

Radiation therapy—A treatment for *leukemia*.

Recall—The ability to remember.

Receptive language—The ability to understand spoken or written communication as well as gestures.

Receptive vocabulary—The words a child is able to understand.

Reciprocal movement—Moving one side of the body and then the other in a coordinated alternate fashion, such as when beating a drum or pedaling a tricycle.

Refraction—The bending of light waves. In vision, the lens bends light rays so that they focus on one point on the *retina*.

Regression—The loss of developmental skills.

Reinforcement—A technique of responding to behavior that is designed to either increase the behavior or decrease it. Reinforcement can be either positive (reward) or negative (punishment).

Related services—Transportation and other developmental, corrective, or supportive services needed to enable a child to benefit from a *special education program*. Under the *IDEA*, a child is entitled to receive these services as part of his *special education* program.

Respiratory infection—An infection, usually viral or bacterial, of the nasal passages, throat, bronchial tubes, or lungs.

Respite care—Care provided to enable parents to have time away from their child with Down syndrome or other disability.

Reward chart—A chart that keeps track of a child's behavior as part of a behavior modification program. The child accumulates points or "stars" on the chart to earn a reward.

Rooting—The instinctive searching for a breast or bottle nipple by a hungry baby.

Rotation (external)—Turning out of the feet, legs, hips, or hands. Seen in babies and children with Down syndrome because of their low muscle tone and joint flexibility.

Section 504 of the Rehabilitation Act—A federal law that prohibits discrimination on the basis of disability in programs receiving federal funds.

Seizure—A sudden loss of consciousness or convulsion resulting from abnormal electrical activity in the brain.

Self-help skills—The ability to take care of one's self, including eating, dressing, bathing, and cleaning. Begins early with awareness, responsiveness, and participation in self-help activities.

Sensory processing—The ability to process sensations, such as touch, sound, light, smell, and movement.

"Separate But Equal"—A repudiated concept used in the past to justify discrimination. The concept held that separate schools for some people (racial minorities and people with disabilities) could be as good as schools the rest of society attended.

Septa (septum)—The wall of cardiac tissue between the chambers of the heart.

Shared risk—An insurance practice of grouping a large number of people together for purposes of spreading insurance risks.

Slanting palpebral fissures—The term describing the upward slanting appearance of the eyes of children with Down syndrome.

Sleep apnea—An interruption in breathing during sleep. A condition in which breathing stops momentarily (for more than 5 seconds) during sleep.

Social skills—The ability to function in groups, to interact with other people.

Social Security Disability Insurance (SSDI)—A federal disability insurance system to provide financial assistance qualified people with disabilities.

Special education—The term commonly used to refer to the education of children with disabilities such as Down syndrome; it includes instruction individually designed to help children with disabilities learn.

Speech language therapist—A therapist trained to work with people to improve their oral motor skills, and to learn both receptive and expressive language.

Sperm—The male reproductive (sex) cell.

Spinal column—The bones that form the spine. The *spinal cord* runs in the middle of this column.

Spinal cord—The nerve tissue that runs up and down the *spinal column.*

SSDI—See *Social Security Disability Insurance.*

SSI—See *Supplemental Security Income.*

Strabismus—Crossed eyes, when one or both eyes look inward or outward.

Standardized test—A test in which a child's performance is compared to the performance of other children of the same age on the same test.

Supplemental Security Income (SSI)—A federal public assistance program for qualified people with disabilities.

Support trust—A trust that requires that funds be expended to pay for the beneficiary's expenses of living, such as housing, food, and transportation.

Supported employment—Employment for people with disabilities that includes some assistance, such as a job coach.

Syndrome—A group of symptoms or traits that indicate a particular condition.

Tactile—Having to do with the sense of touch.

Tactile defensiveness—An overreaction to or avoidance of touch.

Tear ducts—The glands above the eyes that secrete tears.

Therapist—A trained professional who works with children or adults to overcome the effects of developmental problems.

Thyroid—The gland in the neck that secretes the thyroid hormone.

Toddler—A child who is just beginning to walk until about age three.

Tonsils—A small mass of lymph tissue located at the back of the throat.

Tracheo-esophageal fistula—A condition in which there is an abnormal opening between the intestinal tract and respiratory system. This condition requires immediate surgical correction.

Translocation Trisomy 21—A rare form of Down syndrome caused when a part of the extra number-21 chromosome breaks off during meiosis and attaches itself to another chromosome.

Transverse palmar crease—A single crease across the palm of the hands of some children with Down syndrome. One of the physical traits used to identify Down syndrome.

Triple test—A prenatal combined screening for the genetic markers of Down syndrome.

Trisomy—The presence of extra genetic material in the cells; three rather than two chromosomes in the cells.

Tympanometry—A test that measures fluid that may be present behind the ear drum or detects a blockage of the *eustachian tube.*

Ultrasound—The use of high pitched sound waves to create a picture of the inside of a body like that of an X-ray. This procedure is used to examine babies before birth and to help guide medical instruments during *amniocentesis* and *chorionic villus sampling (CVS).*

Umbilical hernia—A protrusion of the navel caused by incomplete muscle development around the navel. Umbilical hernias usually close by themselves.

Uniform Transfers to Minors Act (UTMA)—A law that governs gifts to minors. Under the UTMA, gifts to minors become the property of the minor at age eighteen or twenty-one.

University Affiliated Program (UAP)—A program or clinic associated with a university. These frequently provide medical and developmental services for children with Down syndrome.

University Affiliated Facility (UAF)—See *University Affiliated Program.*

Ventricles—The lower chambers of the heart.

Ventricular septal defect (VSD)—A hole in the wall separating the two lower chambers of the heart.

Vertebrae—The bones of the *spinal column.*

Vestibular—Pertaining to the sensory system located in the inner ear that allows the body to maintain balance and enjoyably participate in movement such as swinging and roughhousing.

Vocational training—Training for specific job skills.

READING LIST

This Reading List is designed especially for parents of children with Down syndrome. The books and pamphlets recommended meet high standards of quality and usefulness.

The Reading List is divided according to the topics covered in each chapter of the book. We have not included books that are outdated or are clinical texts.

This list does not pretend to be complete. There may be many other worthy books available. Check your library and bookstore. Ask other parents and organizations. Please let us know if we have missed a good book or included a bad one.

FOREWORD

Burke, Chris & McDaniel, Jo Beth. *A Special Kind of Hero*. New York: Dell. 1993. Chris Burke, a young man with Down syndrome and co-star of the television series "Life Goes On," tells his life story.

Hunt, Nigel. *The World of Nigel Hunt*. New York: Garrett Publications. 1967. The first personal story written by a person with Down syndrome. Written as a young adult, the book describes his life. Out of print; check your library.

Kingsley, Jason & Levitz, Mitchell. *Count Us In: Growing Up with Down Syndrome*. New York: Harcourt, Brace & Co. 1994. Two men with Down syndrome speak in their own words about their lives, feelings, and hopes for the future.

CHAPTER 1

American Association on Mental Retardation. *Mental Retardation: Definition, Classification, and Systems of Supports*. Washington, DC: American Association on Mental Retardation. 9th edition, 1992. From the organization which establishes the definition of "mental retardation," this book presents the AAMR's revised definition.

Callanan, Charles. *Since Owen: A Parent-to-Parent Guide for Care of the Disabled Child*. Baltimore: The Johns Hopkins University Press. 1990. A guide and personal account about raising a child with disabilities. Well written and useful. Covers many different disabilities.

Cunningham, Cliff. *Down's Syndrome: An Introduction for Parents*. London: Souvenir Press, Ltd. and Cambridge, MA: Brookline Books. 1987. An introduction to Down syndrome published in Great Britain, written by a prominent British Down syndrome specialist.

Dmitriev, Valentine, Ph.D. & Oelwein, Patricia L., MEd., eds. *Advances in Down Syndrome*. Austin, TX: PRO-ED. 1988. A collection of papers by professionals covering a wide range of topics in Down syndrome.

Nadel, Lynn & Rosenthal, Donna, eds. *Down Syndrome: Living and Learning in the Community*. New York: Wiley-Liss. 1995. Publication of papers from the Fifth International Down Syndrome Conference sponsored by the National Down Syndrome Society. Topics range from fostering independence to medical care to supported employment. For parents of younger children, the papers on inclusion and communication skills should be useful.

Pierce, Benjamin A. *The Family Genetic Sourcebook*. New York: John Wiley & Sons, Inc. 1990. A general and basic family guide to genetics and heredity.

Pueschel, Siegfried M., M.D., Ph.D., M.P.H. *A Parent's Guide to Down Syndrome: Toward a Brighter Future*. Baltimore: Paul H. Brookes Publishing Co. 1990. An introduction to Down syndrome, covering birth through adulthood.

Ross, Bette M. *Our Special Child: A Guide To Successful Parenting of Handicapped Children*. New York: Thomas Nelson, Inc. 1993. The personal account of a mother and her son with Down syndrome growing up in California. General information and suggestions.

Smith, Romayne, M.A., CCC-SP. *Children with Mental Retardation: A Parents' Guide*. Bethesda, MD: Woodbine House. 1993. A guide to mental retardation written by both parents and professionals. This book explains diagnosis, causes, medical issues, educational needs, and legal rights.

CHAPTER 2

Buck, Pearl S. *The Child Who Never Grew*. Bethesda, MD: Woodbine House. 1992. A reprint of a classic essay about the famous author's life with her daughter with mental retardation. Includes a Foreword by James Michener and an Introduction by Martha Jablow (see below) written when the book was republished.

Featherstone, Helen. *A Difference in the Family: Living with a Disabled Child*. New York: Penguin Books. 1980. A compassionate look into the emotions of having a child with a disability, based on the author's experiences and interviews with parents and professionals. Highly recommended.

Kanat, Jolie. *Bittersweet Baby*. Minneapolis: CompCare Publishers. 1987. A warm, compassionate, and honest book written by the mother of a baby with Down syndrome about the road toward acceptance of her child.

Kaufman, Sandra Z. *Retarded Isn't Stupid, Mom!* Baltimore: Paul H. Brookes Publishing Co. 1988. A mother's story of her daughter's struggles to live in the community. Her daughter has mental retardation.

Nobel, Vicki. *Down is Up for Aaron Eagle: A Mother's Spiritual Journey with Down's Syndrome.* San Francisco: Harper/San Francisco. 1993. The personal story of the mother of a child with Down syndrome. The author is a shaman— her story is highly spiritual.

Perske, Robert. *Hope for the Families: New Directions for Parents of Persons with Retardation Or Other Disabilities.* Nashville: Abington Press. 1981. A compassionate and philosophical book for parents about adjusting to a child with disabilities.

Simons, Robin. *After the Tears: Parents Talk about Raising a Child with a Disability.* New York: Harcourt, Brace, Jovanovich. 1987. A collection of statements by parents about the emotions of raising a child with a disability.

Spiegle, Jan A. & van den Pol, Richard A. *Making Changes: Family Voices on Living with Disabilities.* Cambridge, MA: Brookline Books. 1993. A collection of essays about the impact of living with a child with disabilities.

Trainer, Marilyn. *Differences in Common: Straight Talk on Mental Retardation, Down Syndrome, and Life.* Bethesda, MD: Woodbine House. 1991. A collection of poignant essays written by the mother of a young man with Down syndrome, spanning his lifetime.

CHAPTER 3

AAUAP, *1994 UAP Resource Guide.* Silver Spring, MD: American Association of University Affiliated Programs (8630 Fenton Street, Suite 410, Silver Spring, MD 20910) 1994. A directory of all University-Affiliated Programs in the United States. These programs often have services for children with Down syndrome.

Batshaw, Mark L., M.D. & Yvonne M. Perret. *Children with Handicaps: A Medical Primer.* Baltimore: Paul H. Brookes Publishing Co. 1992. A layman's medical book about birth defects and other medical conditions of children. Good background reading, but not much information specifically about Down syndrome.

Dox, Ida, Ph.D., Melloni, B. John, Ph.D., Eisner, Gilbert M., M.D. *The Harper-Collins Illustrated Medical Dictionary.* New York: HarperCollins Publishers, Inc. 1993. This illustrated dictionary provides definitions of most common medical terms.

Pueschel, Siegfried M., M.D., Ph.D., M.P.H., Pueschel, Jeanette. *Biomedical Concerns in Persons with Down Syndrome.* Baltimore: Paul H. Brookes Publishing Co. 1992. A technical guide to medical conditions of people with Down syndrome. Recommended for parents with a medical background and for medical professionals.

Van Dyke, D.C., M.D., Mattheis, Philip, M.D., Eberly, Susan, M.A., Williams, Janet, R.N. *Medical and Surgical Care for Children with Down Syndrome: A Guide for Parents.* Bethesda, MD: Woodbine House. 1995. A guide for parents about the medical concerns of children with Down syndrome.

CHAPTER 4

Finston, Peggy, M.D. *Parenting Plus: Raising Children with Special Health Needs.* New York: Dutton. 1990. A basic guide to general health and disability issues.

Lansky, Vicki. *Toilet Training.* New York: Bantam Books, Inc. 1984. A parents' guide to toilet training children. Useful information, but not focused on toilet training children with disabilities.

Mack, Alison. *Toilet Learning: The Picture Book Technique for Children and Parents.* Boston: Little, Brown & Co. 1978. A comprehensive toilet training method, written in two parts for parents and children.

Satter, Ellyn, R.D. *Child of Mine: Feeding with Love and Good Sense.* Palo Alto, CA: Bull Publishing Company. 1983. A useful book about your child's diet and nutrition.

Satter, Ellyn, R.D. *How to Get Your Kid to Eat...But Not Too Much.* Palo Alto, CA: Bull Publishing Company. 1987. This book describes how to balance your child's nutritional needs.

Segal, Marilyn, Ph.D. *In Time and With Love.* New York: Newmarket Press. 1988. A general guide to parenting a child with a disability, written by a mother and professional. It includes some information about Down syndrome.

CHAPTER 5

Anderson, Rachel. *The Bus People.* New York: Henry Holt and Company, Inc. 1989. Recommended for older siblings (middle and high school) and parents, this collection of stories is written from the standpoint of several young people with different disabilities, including Down syndrome.

Briggs, Dorothy Corkille. *Your Child's Self-Esteem.* New York: Doubleday & Co., 1975. A parents' guide to building a child's self-esteem and feelings of self-worth.

Bunnett, Rochelle. *Friends in the Park.* New York: Checkerboard Press, Inc. 1993. A children's picture book about the children in a park. Some have disabilities and some do not, but all play together.

Cairo, Shelley. *Our Brother Has Down's Syndrome: An Introduction for Children.* Toronto: Annick Press, Ltd. 1985. An excellent book to help parents introduce young siblings to Down syndrome. Highly recommended.

Dodds, Bill. *My Sister Annie.* Honesdale, PA: Boyds Mill Press, Inc. 1993. Recommended for children between the 4th and 8th grades, this novel presents many of the emotions and feelings siblings of children with Down syndrome may have.

Dougan, Terrell, Lyn Isbell, Patricia Vyas, comps. *We Have Been There: A Guidebook for Families of People with Mental Retardation.* Nashville: Abingdon Press. 1983. A collection of short inspiring stories of families coping with children with mental retardation. Out of print, but worth checking for at your library.

Dwight, Laura. *We Can Do It.* New York: Checkerboard Press, Inc. 1992. A children's book about the things children with disabilities *can* do.

Featherstone, Helen. *A Difference in the Family: Living with a Disabled Child.* New York: Penguin Books. 1980. A compassionate look into the emotions of having a child with a disability, based on the author's experiences and interviews with parents and professionals. Highly recommended.

Jablow, Martha. *Cara: Growing with a Retarded Child.* Philadelphia: Temple University Press. 1982. The personal account of the childhood of a girl with Down syndrome, told by her mother, a journalist.

Jones, Ron. *The Acorn People.* New York: Bantam. 1990. The endearing story of a summer camp for children with different disabilities.

Klein, Stanley & Schleifer, Maxwell. *It Isn't Fair: Siblings of Children with Disabilities.* Greenwood. 1993. A collection of articles from *Exceptional Parent* magazine about siblings of children with disabilities.

Lobato, Debra. *Brothers, Sisters, and Special Needs: Information and Activities for Helping Young Siblings of Children with Chronic Illnesses and Developmental Disabilities.* Baltimore: Paul H. Brookes Publishing Co. 1990. A guide to information and activities for siblings of children with special needs.

Marsh, Jayne & Boggis, Carol. *From the Heart: On Being the Mother of a Child with Special Needs.* Bethesda, MD: Woodbine House. 1995. Nine mothers explore the emotional terrain of raising children with special needs, including Down syndrome.

Meyer, Donald J., Vadasy, Patricia F., & Fewell, Rebecca R. *Living with a Brother or Sister with Special Needs.* Seattle, WA: University of Washington Press. 1985. A book written for children about having a sibling with a disability.

Meyer, Donald. *Uncommon Fathers: Reflections on Raising a Child with a Disability.* Bethesda, MD: Woodbine House. 1995. A collection of essays about the experience of being the father of a child with special needs. Includes several essays written by fathers of children with Down syndrome.

Miller, Nancy B., Ph.D. *Nobody's Perfect: Living and Growing with Children Who Have Special Needs.* A guide to the emotions and adjustments of having a child with a disability in the family.

Perske, Robert. *New Life In The Neighborhood: How Persons with Retardation Or Other Disabilities Can Help Make a Good Community Better.* Nashville: Abingdon Press. 1980. A compassionate and philosophical look at people with disabilities in the community, illustrated beautifully.

Perske, Robert. *Show Me No Mercy: A Compelling Story of Remarkable Courage.* Nashville: Abingdon Press. 1984. A novel about a father and his son with Down syndrome, written by the author of several nonfiction books about people with mental retardation.

Powell, Thomas H. & Gallagher, Peggy A. *Brothers & Sisters—A Special Part of Exceptional Families.* Baltimore: Paul H. Brookes Publishing Co. 1993. A detailed, yet clinical, examination of the siblings of exceptional children. The book primarily reviews research on the subject.

Rabe, Berniece. *Where's Chimpy?* Morton Grove, IL: Albert Whitman & Co. 1988. A bedtime storybook about Misty's (who has Down syndrome) search for her stuffed animal, Chimpy. Recommended.

Schleifer, Maxwell J. & Stanley D. Klein, eds. *The Disabled Child and The Family: An Exceptional Parent Reader.* Boston: The Exceptional Parent Press. 1985. A collection of articles from "Exceptional Parent" magazine covering a wide range of topics related to having a person with disabilities in the family.

Sullivan, Tom. *Special Parent, Special Child: Parents of Children with Disabilities Share Their Trials, Triumphs, and Hard-Won Wisdom.* New York: G.P. Putnam's Sons. 1995. Interviews with families with children with disabilities (including Down syndrome).

Thompson, Mary. *My Brother, Matthew.* Bethesda, MD: Woodbine House. 1992. An illustrated children's book written from the perspective of a sibling of a child with a disability (not specified).

Turnbull, H. Rutherford & Turnbull, Ann P. *Parents Speak Out: Then And Now.* New York: MacMillan. 1985. A collection of articles by parents of children with mental retardation, focusing on how families learned to cope.

Westridge Young Writers Workshop. *Kids Explore the Gifts of Children with Special Needs.* Santa Fe, NM: John Muir Publications. 1994. A collection of stories of children with disabilities told by their classmates. Included is a story about a child with Down syndrome.

CHAPTER 6

Kumin, Libby, Ph.D. *Communication Skills in Children with Down Syndrome: A Guide for Parents.* Bethesda, MD: Woodbine House. 1994. This guide for parents explains language development in children with Down syndrome and how parents can help encourage good development. Contains activities.

White, Burton L. *The First Three Years of Life.* Revised Edition. New York: Prentice Hall Press. 1985. One of the classics of childhood development, covering the first three years of life.

CHAPTER 7

Coleman, Jeanine. *The Early Intervention Dictionary: A Multidisciplinary Guide to Terminology.* Bethesda, MD: Woodbine House. 1993. A guide to the terminology used in early intervention.

Dmitriev, Valentine, Ph.D. *Time To Begin: Early Education for Children with Down Syndrome.* Milton, Washington: Caring, Inc. 1982. A handbook for early infant stimulation for babies with Down syndrome, covering activities in all areas of development during the first years of life.

Hanson, Marci J. *Teaching Your Down's Syndrome Infant: A Guide for Parents and Professionals.* Austin, TX: PRO-ED. 1987. A useful guide for parents and professionals to early infant education. Provides lesson plans for all areas of infant development.

Mannix, Darlene. *Social Skills Activities for Special Children.* New York: The Center for Applied Research in Education. 1993. A collection of lessons and activities to help young children learn social behavior skills.

McConkey, Roy & Jeffree, Dorothy. *Making Toys for Handicapped Children.* Englewood Cliffs, NJ: Prentice-Hall, Inc., 1983. A guide make and use toys suited to children with disabilities.

National Down Syndrome Society. *Inclusion.* New York: National Down Syndrome Society. 1995. A booklet that introduces inclusive education and stresses the elements needed for a successful inclusion program.

Oelwein, Patricia L. *Teaching Reading to Children with Down Syndrome: A Guide for Parents and Teachers.* Bethesda, MD: Woodbine House. 1995. This guide presents a program specifically designed for teaching children with Down syndrome to read.

Rosenberg, Michael, Ph.D. & Edmond-Rosenberg, Irene. *The Special Education Sourcebook: A Teacher's Guide to Programs, Materials, and Information Sources.* Bethesda, MD: Woodbine House. 1994. A book of sources for resources and information about special education. Primarily written for professionals, but useful to parents also.

Rynders, John E. & Horrobin, J. Margaret. *Down Syndrome: Birth to Adulthood— Giving Families an Edge.* Denver, CO: Love Publishing Co. 1995. This introduction to Down syndrome contains a lot of information about education and inclusion.

Schwartz, Sue & Miller, Joan Heller. *The Language of Toys.* Bethesda, MD: Woodbine House. 1988. This book explains language development and the use of toys to encourage good language development.

CHAPTER 8

Anderson, Winifred, Stephen Chitwood, Deidre Hayden. *Negotiating The Special Education Maze: A Guide for Parents and Teachers.* Bethesda, MD: Woodbine House. 1990. A guide to helping parents get the best special education for their child through advocacy.

ARC National Insurance And Benefits Committee. *How To Provide for Their Future.* Arlington, TX: The Arc. 1984. A booklet that explains many of the concerns about wills, estate planning, insurance, and government benefits for parents of children with mental retardation.

Beckman, Paula J. & Beckman, Gayle B. *Deciphering the System: A Guide for Families of Young Children with Disabilities.* Cambridge, MA: Brookline Books. 1993. A parents' guide to the IDEA and how to get the most from the law for your child.

Cutler, Barbara Coyne. *You, Your Child, and "Special" Education: A Guide to Making the System Work.* Baltimore: Paul H. Brookes Publishing Co. 1993. A guide to special education law, rights, and procedures.

Des Jardins, Charlotte. *How To Get Services By Being Assertive.* Chicago: Family Resource Center on Disabilities. 1980. A handbook for obtaining services for children with disabilities. Contains suggestions on advocating for your child.

Des Jardins, Charlotte. *How To Organize an Effective Parent Advocacy Group and Move Bureaucracies.* Chicago: Family Resource Center on Disabilities. 1980. A handbook on organizing parent advocacy groups and working for change in educational services for children with disabilities.

Moore, Ralph J., Jr. *Handbook On Estate Planning for Families of Developmentally Disabled Persons in Maryland, The District of Columbia and Virginia.* Baltimore: Maryland State Planning Council On Developmental Disabilities. 1981. A guide to estate planning for parents of exceptional children. Although written for the laws of two states and the District of Columbia, the general legal principles are generally applicable.

Parent Advocacy Coalition for Educational Rights (PACER). *The ADA: A Guide for People with Disabilities, Their Families and Advocates.* Minneapolis: PACER Center, Inc., 4826 Chicago Avenue, Minneapolis, MN 55417–1098, 612/827–2966. 1993. A concise overview of the ADA written for non-lawyers.

Russell, L. Mark, J.D. *Planning for the Future.* Evanston, IL: American Publishing Co. 1993. A guide to estate planning, guardianship, wills, and financial planning for parents of children with disabilities.

United States Department of Education. *"To Assure The Free Appropriate Public Education of All Children with Disabilities:" Sixteenth Annual Report to Congress On the Implementation of The Individuals with Disabilities Education Act.* Office of Special Education and Rehabilitative Services, United States Department of Education. 1994. The annual report about the IDEA, and what is being done, or not being done, to carry out its purpose.

United States Equal Employment Opportunity Commission, United States Department of Justice, Civil Rights Division. *The Americans with Disabilities Act: Questions and Answers.* 1992. A useful booklet that explains the basic terms of the ADA.

Magazines and Journals

Down Syndrome News. National Down Syndrome Congress, 1605 Chantilly Rd., Atlanta, GA 30324. The official newsletter of the National Down Syndrome Congress, published ten times a year. One of the best publications for parents, filled with information and news. Available to members.

The Exceptional Parent. Psy-Ed Corporation. P.O. Box 3000, Denville, NJ 07834, 800/247–8080 (subscriptions) A useful and informative magazine for parents of children with a wide variety of disabilities. Highly recommended for parents.

People With Special Needs/Down Syndrome Report. 1409 North First Street, Aberdeen, South Dakota 57401. (E-Mail: robjohns@sendit.nodak.edu). Published by a father and son (who has Down syndrome), this newsletter covers topics in Down syndrome.

RESOURCE GUIDE

This resource guide contains references to a wide variety of organizations that can help parents of babies with Down syndrome. We wish to thank the National Down Syndrome Congress and the National Information Center for Children and Youth with Disabilities (NICHCY) for contributing much of the information in this Guide.

The following list briefly describes the different types of organizations listed in this Resource Guide:

• **State Department of Education**—The state agency or agencies responsible for providing special education, including early intervention to children with Down syndrome. In many states, the Department of Education administers both early intervention services (birth through age two) and services for pre-school and school aged children. When different agencies administer these programs, both agencies are listed.

• **Protection & Advocacy Service**—Legal organizations established to protect the rights of people with disabilities, including children with Down syndrome. They can supply information about the educational, health, residential, social, and legal services available for children with Down syndrome.

• **The Arc (formerly the Association for Retarded Citizens)**—Each state's Arc is listed, but there are many local (city and county) branches. These local organizations and their many programs are essential resources for parents. They can provide information and referral, put you in touch with other parents, and provide respite care. To find The Arc nearest you, check with your state Arc.

• **University Affiliated Programs**—There are many programs that are affiliated with universities that offer developmental services to parents of children with Down syndrome and other disabilities.

• **Parent Information and Training Centers**—Established and funded by federal law, these centers provide information and training to parents in how to use the IDEA and other laws for their child's education.

• **Organizations**—There are many different types of organization that can help parents of children with Down syndrome. These include parent support groups, local organizations affiliated with national Down syndrome organizations, and information sources. To get the most up-to-date listing, call NICHCY at their toll-free number.

National Organizations

American Association of University Affiliated Programs for
  Persons with Developmental Disabilities
8630 Fenton Street
Suite 410
Silver Spring, MD 20910
301/588–8252
Many universities offer programs and services for children with disabilities, including Down syndrome. These services can include developmental & health clinics for children with Down syndrome and early intervention. For the location of the University Affiliated Program nearest you, contact the AAUAP.

American Speech-Language-Hearing Association
10801 Rockville Pike
Rockville, MD 20852
301/897–5700 (Voice/TDD).
ASHA researches communication disorders and is the national organization for speech and language therapists. ASHA offers brochures on speech and hearing disorders and information about computer software and augmentative communication systems.

The Arc (formerly the Association for Retarded Citizens)
National Headquarters
500 East Border Street
Suite 300
P.O. Box 300649
Arlington, TX 76010
817/261–6003
A grassroots national organization that advocates on behalf of people with mental retardation and other disabilities. Publishes information about all types of disabilities and supports an extensive network of local affiliates.

Association for the Care of Children's Health
7910 Woodmont Avenue
Suite 300
Bethesda, MD 20814
301/654–6549
301/986–4553 (FAX)
Through education, advocacy, and research, ACCH increases awareness of psychological and developmental needs of children with chronic illnesses or disabilities. ACCH offers a bi-monthly newsletter and Parent Resource Guide, as well as other publications.

Canadian Association for Community Living
4700 Keele Street
Kinsman Building
North York, ON Canada M3J 1P3
416/661–9611
416/661–5701 (FAX)
This national organization provides similar services for people with disabilities in Canada as The Arc provides in the United States.

Canadian Down Syndrome Society
811 14th Street, NW
Calgary, AB Canada T2N 2A4
403/270–8500
403/270–8291
This organization advocates for people with Down syndrome, provides information to
parents, and sponsors conferences.

Clearinghouse on Disability Information
Office of Special Education and Rehabilitation Services
U.S. Department of Education
400 Maryland Avenue, SW
Room 3132, Switzer Building
Washington, DC 20202–2524
202/205–8241
This federal organization offers information on civil rights, federal benefits, medical serv-
ices, and support organizations. It publishes *Pocket Guide to Federal Help for Individuals with
Disabilities.*

Council for Exceptional Children
1920 Association Drive
Reston, VA 22091–1589
703/620–3660
This organization represents special education teachers nationally. It focuses on the educational needs of children with disabilities. It conducts computer searches for information about the education of children with disabilities and publishes several journals.

ERIC Clearinghouse on Handicapped and Gifted Children
Council for Exceptional Children
1920 Association Drive
Reston, VA 22091–1589
This clearinghouse provides information about the education and development of students who have disabilities, including early intervention. Conducts online database
searches.

National Association of Protection and Advocacy Systems
900 Second Street, NE
Suite 211
Washington, DC 20002
202/408–9514
202/408–9520 (FAX)
E-Mail: HN4537@handsnet.org
This is the national association for all state Protection and Advocacy offices. It can refer
you to the nearest P & A office.

National Down Syndrome Congress
7000 Peachtree-Dunwoody Rd., NE
Building 5, Suite 100
Atlanta, GA 30328
800/232-NDSC
E-mail: NDSCCenter@aol.com
Website: www.ndsccenter.org
A national organization of parents and professionals. The NDSC publishes "Down Syn-
drome News" and "Down Syndrome Headline News" (written by and for people with
Down syndrome), holds an annual convention, provides information and referral through

its toll-free number, and coordinates an extensive national network of local affiliates. Information sheets and booklets available. An excellent resource.

National Down Syndrome Society
666 Broadway
New York, NY 10012
800/221–4602
212/979–2873 (FAX)
A national organization that works to promote a better understanding of people with Down syndrome. The NDSS publishes a quarterly newsletter and "News and Views" (a publication for people with Down syndrome), sponsors scientific and educational research into Down syndrome, and sponsors scientific conferences. Booklets and information sheets available.

National Information Center for Children and Youth with Disabilities (NICHCY)
P.O. Box 1492
Washington, DC 20013–1492
800/695–0285
202/884–8441 (FAX)
E-Mail: nichy@capcon.net
An extremely valuable resource for parents, NICHCY provides free information to parents of children with disabilities. NICHCY specializes in providing information about state and local resources. For example, if you want to know who to contact in your state about early intervention, NICHCY can tell you. Ask for their "State Sheet" for your state. In addition, NICHCY has information sheets on a wide range of disability topics.

National Parent Network on Disabilities
1600 Prince Street
Suite 115
Alexandria, VA 22314
703/684–6763
703/836–1232 (FAX)
E-Mail: npnd@aol.com
This national organization advocates on behalf of parents of children with disabilities. It also provides information to parents about government policy affecting people with disabilities.

National Parent-to-Parent Support and Information System
P.O. Box 907
Blue Ridge, GA 30513
800/651–1151
706/632–8830 (FAX)
E-Mail: judd103w@wonder.em.cdc.gov
This is the national organization for all Parent-to-Parent groups, a national network of parent support groups. Call to find the Parent-to-Parent group nearest you.

Senate Document Room
Hart Building
Washington, DC 20515
202/228-2815 (FAX)
You can obtain a copy of any federal bill or law, including IDEA or the ADA, by contacting this office. Requests must be submitted by fax, by mail, or in person (not by phone).

Sibling Information Network
The A.J. Pappanikou Center on Special Education and Rehabilitation
62 Washington Street
Middletown, CT 06457
203/344–7500
203/344–7595 (FAX)
This is an organization for siblings of people with disabilities. Its quarterly newsletter contains resources and information concerning family issues.

Sibling Support Project
P.O. Box 5371, CL-09
Seattle, WA 98105–0371
206/368–4911
206/368–4816 (FAX)
This organization provides workshops and training to parents and professionals about sibling issues.

Special Olympics
1325 G Street, NW
Suite 500
Washington, DC 20005
202/628–3630
202/824–0200 (FAX)
An international program of physical fitness, sports training, and athletic competition for children and adults with disabilities. Open to competitors of all ages and ability levels.

ALABAMA

AL Dept. of Educ, Div of Special Education Services
PO Box 302101
Montgomery, AL 36130–2101
205/242–8114
800/392–8020(in AL)
Contact: Bill East, Director

Early Intervention Program
Department of Rehabilitation Services
2129 East South Blvd., PO Box 11586
Montgomery, AL 36111–0586
205/281–8780
Contact: Ouida Holder, Part H Coordinator

Alabama Disabilities Advocacy Program (ADAP)
The University of Alabama, PO Box 870395
Tuscaloosa, AL 35487–0395
205/348–4928

Contact: Reuben Cook, Director

The ARC of Alabama
444 South Decatur Street
Montgomery, AL 36104
205/262–7688
Contact: Elizabeth Prince, Executive Director

Civitan International Research Center and Sparks Clinic
University of AL at Birmingham
1720 Seventh Avenue South
Birmingham, AL 35233
205/934–5471
Contact: Craig T. and Sharon L. Ramey, Directors

Special Education Action Committee Inc. (SEAC)
PO Box 161274
Mobile, AL 36616–2274
205/478–1208

800/222–7322 (in AL)
Contact: Carol Blades, Director

Huntsville Down Syndrome Association
1075 Dockside Drive #907
Huntsville, AL 35824–1413
205/882–0484
Contact: Beverly Basoglu

The Association for Down Syndrome Citizens
3408 Wellborne Dr. E.
Mobile, AL 36695
205/661–1920
Contact: Paul & Gene Connolly

ALASKA

Office of Special Education/AK Department of Education
801 West 10th St., Suite 200
Juneau, AK 99801–1894
907/465–2971
Contact: Myra Howe, Director

Early Intervention Services/Infant Learning Program
State Department of Health & Social Services
1231 Gambell Street
Anchorage, AK 99501–4627
Contact: Pam Muth

Advocacy Services of Alaska
615 East 82nd, Suite 101
Anchorage, AK 99518
907/344–1002
Contact: Rick Tessandore, Director

Special Education Parent Resource Center
2220 Nichols Street
Anchorage, AK 99508
907/263–9285
Contact: Kim Crews

Arc of Anchorage
2211–A Arca Drive
Anchorage, AK 99506
907/277–6677
Contact: Mary Jane Starlings

Alaska Chapter National Down Syndrome Congress
HC 83 Box 1706
Eagle River, AK 99577
907/694–2545
Contact: Donna Davidson

P.A.R.E.N.T.S., Inc.
540 W. Int'l Airport Road, Suite 200
Anchorage, AK 99518
800/478–7678 (V/TTY)
907/563–2246
Contact: Jenny Weaver

PARENTS
Box 32198
Juneau, AK 99803
800/478–7678
907/790–2246
Contact: Judie Ebbert Rich

Caring Hearts
2768 Triplehorn Lane
Fairbanks, AK 99709
907/455–6529
Contact: Sat Dharan Khalsa

ARIZONA

Special Education Section, Department of Education
1535 West Jefferson
Phoenix, AZ 85007
602/542–3084
Contact: Kay Lund, Director

Special Education Section, Department of Education
1535 West Jefferson
Phoenix, AZ 85007
602/542–3852
Contact: Lynn Busenbark, Preschool Coordinator

Arizona Center for Law in the Public Interest
3724 N. 3rd St., Suite 30
Phoenix, AZ 85012
602/274–6287
Contact: Anne Ronan, Staff Attorney

The Arc of Arizona
5610 South Central
Phoenix, AZ 85040
602/243–1787
800/252–9054
Contact: Richard Young, Exec Director

Pilot Parents Partnerships
2150 East Highland Avenue, #105
Phoenix, AZ 85016
602/468–3001
800/237–3007 (in AZ)
Contact: Mary Slaughter, Exec. Director

SHARING-Down Syndrome Support & Information Network
2451 W. Paradise Lane
Phoenix, AZ 85023
602/993–2229
602/275–1426
Contact: Nancy Margan/Anita Chavez

Forward Challenge
1810 Hazelwood Lane
Prescott, AZ 86301
602/776–1277
Contact: Therese McLoughlin

ARKANSAS

Preschool Programs, Special Education, Dept. of Educ
#4 Capitol Mall, Room 105–C
Little Rock, AR 72201–1071
501/682–4222
Contact: Sandra K. Reifeiss, Coordinator

Div. of Dev. Dis. Svcs. Dept of Human Services
PO Box 1437, Donaghey Plaza, North 5th Floor, Slot 2520
Little Rock, AR 72203–1437
501/682–8676
Contact: Jackie Barentine, Part H Coordinator

Advocacy Services, Inc.
1100 N. University, Suite 201
Little Rock, AR 72207
501/296–1775
800/482–1174(V/TDD)
Contact: Nan Ellen East, Exec. Director

The Arc of Arkansas
2725 Cantrell, Suite 203
Little Rock, AR 72202
501/664–5553
800/264–5553
Contact: Cynthia Stone, Exec. Director

University of AR, University Affiliated Program
1120 Marshall, Suite 306
Little Rock, AR 72202
501/370–3760
Contact: Mark Swanson, MD Director

Arkansas Disability Coalition
10002 West Markham, Suite B-7

Little Rock, AR 72205
501/221–1330 (V/TDD)
800/223–1330 (V/TDD)
Contact: Bonnie Johnson, Director

Parent-to-Parent
The ARC of Arkansas
2725 Cantrell, Suite 203
Little Rock, AR 72202
501/664–5553
800/264–5553
Contact: Brenda Reed, Coordinator

Down Syndrome Parents of Western Arkansas
PO Box 4745
Fort Smith, AR 72914–4745
501/783–3991
Contact: Norma Lucas

Richardson Center
1760 Woodland
Fayetteville, AR 72703
501/449–4420
Contact: Dr. Janice Hardin

Down Syndrome Families and Friends
Box 193812
Little Rock, AR 72219–3812
501/562–1470
Contact: Becky Singleton

CALIFORNIA

Special Education, Department of Education
515 L Street, Suite 270
Sacramento, CA 95814
916/445–4729
Contact: Leo D. Sandoval, Director

Early Start Program
1600 9th Street, Room #310
Sacramento, CA 95814
916/654–2773
Contact: Julie Jackson, Manager

Protection & Advocacy, Inc.
100 Howe Avenue, Suite 185N
Sacramento, CA 95825
916/488–9950
800/776–5746 (in CA)
Contact: Catherine Blakemore, Exec. Director

Arc CA
120 I Street, 2nd Floor

Sacramento, CA 95814
916/552–6619
Contact: Gary A. Tonis, Exec Director

Team of Advocates for Special Kids
(TASK)
100 West Cerritos Avenue
Anaheim, CA 92805–6546
714/533–TASK
Contact: Joan Tellefsen, Director

Down Syndrome League
2964 Miranda Avenue
Alamo, CA 94507
510/743–1792
Contact: Martha Hogan/Janet Richmond

Down Syndrome Parent Group of Kern
8008 Dottie Court
Bakersfield, CA 93308
805/832–7964
Contact: Sheri Bryant

Keeping Informed on Down Syndrome
PO Box 6800, Suite 254
Corona, CA 91718
909/371–5800
Contact: Janine & Mark Macias

Exceptional Parents Unlimited Down Syndrome Network
4120 N. First Street
Fresno, CA 93726
209/229–2000
Contact: Leslie Lee

Irvine Childrens Educational Center
5120 Bonita Canyon Road
Irvine, CA 92715
714/854–7600
Contact: Pam Sears

Project Cope
Ontario-Pomona ARC
8939 Vernon, Suite H
Montclair, CA 91763
714/985–3116
Contact: Mary Jean Mauney

Down Syndrome Association of Los Ange-
les Inc.
8949 Reseda Blvd.
Suite 109
Northridge, CA 91324–3943
800/464–8995
818/718–6363
Contact: Nancy Hall

PROUD
Box 5822
Orange, CA 92668
714/974–6419
Contact: Amy Braun & Joyce Taylor

Parents of Down Syndrome of Northern
CA
1127 Hilltop Drive
Redding, CA 96003
916/223–3120
Contact: Sharon Chestnut

Padres of Personas con Sindrome Down
Box 1695
Reseda, CA 91337
213/254–7834
Contact: Juan Gonzalez

Sacramento Area DS Association
1228 La Sierra Drive
Sacramento, CA 95864
916/483–1110
Contact: Teresa Androvich

Down Syndrome Association of San Diego
Box 881883
San Diego, CA 92168–0038
619/571–7001
Contact: Betty Cabral

Support for Parents with Special Children
2601 Mission St., Ste 710
San Francisco, CA 94110
415/282–7494
415/346–6858
Contact: Kathy Darby

PODS/Parents Helping Parents
535 Race St.
Suite 220
San Jose, CA 95126
408/727-5775
Contact: Maria Larcher

Down Syndrome Network of SLO County
2594 Black Walnut Road
San Luis Obispo, CA 93405
805/595–9529
Contact: Pam Kennedy

Peninsula Down Syndrome Association of
PARCA
1650 Amphlette Blvd.
Suite 213

San Mateo, CA 94402
415/312–0730
Contact: Margaret Jesch & Sue Dig

Down Syndrome Parents, Teachers and Friends, Inc.
Box 6443
Santa Maria, CA 93456
805/937–2465
Contact: Joanne Cargill

South Bay Down Syndrome Parents Support Group
21515 Hawthorne Blvd.
Suite 211
Torrance, CA 90503
213/375–6050
Contact: Marcia Good

Solano Parents United for Down Syndrome
707 Tuolumne Street
Vallejo, CA 94590
707/552–2935
Contact: Carol Gonsalves

Ventura County Down Syndrome Association
Easter Seal Society
10730 Henderson Road
Ventura, CA 93004
805/647–1147
Contact: Jane Bonn

Up for Down
510 E. Ghent St.
San Dimas, CA 91773
909/592–3216
Contact: Caroline Parikh

KIDS
39335 Chalfont Lane
Palmdale, CA 93551
805/267–6450
Contact: Roberta Dunn

COLORADO

Spec. Ed. Svcs. Unit/CO Dept of Educ
201 East Colfax Avenue
Denver, CO 80203
303/866–6695
Contact: Fred Smokoski, Director

Early Childhood Initiatives
State Department of Education
201 East Colfax, Room, 301
Denver, CO 80203

303/866–6709
Contact: April Block, Part H Coordinator

The Legal Center
455 Sherman Street, Suite 130
Denver, CO 80203
303/722–0300
800/288–1376
Contact: Mary Anne Harvery, Exec Director

John F. Kennedy Center for Developmental Disabilities
University of CO Health Sciences Center
4200 East Ninth Avenue, Box C-234
Denver, CO 80262
303/270–7224
Contact: Cordelia Robinson, Director

PEAK Parent Center, Inc.
6055 Lehman Drive, Suite 101
Colorado Springs, CO 80918
719/531–9400
800/284–0251 (In CO and TDD)
Contact: Judy Martz & Barbara Buswell

Colorado Springs Down Syndrome Association
Box 2364
Colorado Springs, CO 80901
719/633–1133
Contact: Patricia A. Haug

Mile High Down Syndrome Association
Box 620847
Littleton, CO 80162
303/797–1699
Contact: Linda Barth

CONNECTICUT

Bureau of Early Childhood Education & Social Svcs.
CT Department of Education
25 Industrial Park Road
Middletown, CT 06457
203/638–4205
Contact: Kay Halverson, Coordinator

Early Childhood Unit
CT Department of Education
25 Industrial Park Road
Middletown, CT 06457
203/638–4208
Contact: Joan Brinckerhoff, Birth -3 Part H Coordinator

Office of P&A for Persons with Disabilities
60 B Weston Street
Hartford, CT 06120–1551
203/297–4300
800/842–7303 (in CT)
Contact: Eliot J. Dober, Exec Director

Arc CT
1030 New Britian Avenue, Suite 102B
West Hartford, CT 06110
203/953–8335
Contact: Margaret Dignoti, Exec Director

A.J. Pappanikou Ctr. on Spec Educ &
Rehabilitation, A University Affiliated
Program
62 Washington Street
Middletown, CT 06457
203/344–7500
Contact: Orv. C. Karan, Director

Connecticut Parent Advocacy Center
(CPAC)
5 Church Lane, Suite 4
PO Box 579
East Lyme, CT 06333
203/739–3089
800/445–2722 (in CT)
Contact: Nancy Prescott, Director

WeCAHR
11 Lake Avenue Ext
Danbury, CT 06811
203/792–3540
Contact: Pat Tomka, Coordinator

Connecticut Down Syndrome Congress,
Inc.
Box 951
Cheshire, CT 06410
203/250–1223
Contact: Linda Ruggiero

LOVARH
1 Hartford Avenue
Old Saybrook, CT 06475
203/388–3803
Contact: George D. Duryea

The Family Center/Newington Children's
Hospital
181 E. Cedar Street
Newington, CT 06111
203/667–5288

DELAWARE

Management Svcs Division
Health and Social Services, 2nd Floor,
Room 231
1901 North DuPont Highway
New Castle, DE 19720
302/577–4647
Contact: Nancy Wilson, Part H Coordina-
tor

Disabilities Law Program
144 East Market Street
Georgetown, DE 19947
302/856–0038
Contact: Pat Shipe, Administrator

Arc of Delaware
240 North James Street, Suite B-2
Wilmington, DE 19804
302/996–9400
Contact: Rita Mariani-Smith, Exec Director

Parent Information Center of DE, Inc.
(PIC)
700 Barksdale Road, Suite 6
Newark, DE 19711
302/366–0152
302/366–0178 (TDD)
Contact: Marie-Anne Aghazadian, Exec Director

Down Syndrome Association of Delaware
Inc.
3 Hummock Court
Wilmington, DE 19803
302/762–4747
Contact: Mary Ann Evans, President

DISTRICT OF COLUMBIA

State Office of Spec. Educ/Browne Administrative Unit
26th Street & Benning Road, NE
Washington, DC 20002
202/724–4178
Contact: Lila Vanderhorst, Asst Director

Commission on Social Services
Department of Human Services
609 H St., NE 4th Floor
Washington, DC 20002
202/727–3755
Contact: Sharman Dennis, Part H Coordinator

Logan Child Study Center
3rd and G Streets, NE
Washington, DC 20002
202/724-4800

Information, P&A Center for People with Disabilities (IPACHI)
4455 Connecticut Avenue, NW Suite B-100
Washington, DC 20008
202/966-8081
202/966-2500 (TDD)
Contact: Vivianne Hardy-Townes, Exec Director

District of Columbia ARC
900 Varnum Street, NE
Washington, DC 20017
202/636-2950
Contact: Shirley Wade, Exec Director

Creating Opportunities for Parent Empowerment (COPE)
810 Potomac Avenue SE 1st Floor Rear
Washington, DC 20003
202/543-6482
800/515-2673
Contact: Charlene Howard, Director

District of Columbia Down Syndrome Association
4907 16th Street, NE
Washington, DC 20017
202/526-5225
Contact: Rebecca Forsyth

FLORIDA

Bur. of Educ for Exceptional Students
Dept of Educ
325 West Gaines Street, Suite 614
Tallahassee, FL 32399-0400
904/488-1570
Contact: Bettye D. Weir, Bureau Chief

Office of Early Intervention & School Readiness
Division of Public Schools/Dept of Education
325 West Gaines Street, Suite 754
Tallahassee, FL 32399-0400
904/488-6830
Contact: Nancy D. Thomas, Program Specialist

Advocacy Center for Persons with Disabilities
2671 Executive Center Circle West, Suite 100
Tallahassee, FL 32301-5024
904/488-9071
Contact: Marcia Beach, Exec Director

Arc FL
411 East College Avenue
Tallahassee, FL 32301
904/921-0460
Contact: Chris Schuh

Mailman Center for Child Development
University of Miami School of Medicine
PO Box 016820-D-820
Miami, FL 33101
305/547-6635
Contact: Robert Stempfel, MD Director

Family Network on Disabilities of FL, Inc
5510 Gray St., Suite 220
Tampa, FL 33609
813/289-1122
800/825-5736
Contact: Janet Jacoby, Exec Director

Gold Coast Down Syndrome Organization, Inc.
22626 SW 65 Terrace
Boca Raton, FL 33428
407/451-2163
Contact: Terri Harmon

Down Syndrome Support Group of Lee County, Inc.
12995 S. Cleveland Avenue
Suite 103BB
Ft. Meyers, FL 33907
813/549-0877
Contact: June De Long

Broward County Gold Coast Down Organization
10691 London Street
Cooper City, FL 33026
407/432-1009
Contact: Mitchell & Susan Holeve

Parents of Down Syndrome
5555 Biscayne Blvd.
3rd Floor
Miami, FL 33127
305/759-8500
Contact: Sylvia Sanchez

Central Florida Down Syndrome Association
2600 E. Jackson Street
Orlando, FL 32803
407/894–8401
Contact: Denise L. Duffey

Space Coast Early Intervention Center, Inc.
2524 Palm Bay Road, NE
Suite A
Palm Bay, FL 32905
407/729–6858
Contact: Betsy Farmer

Down Association of Jacksonville
4810 Otter Creek Lane
Ponte Vedra Beach, FL 32082
904/285–5904
Contact: Laura Watts

Up With Downs of Pinellas County
912 Toddsmill Trace
Tarpon Springs, FL 34689
813/937–6555
Contact: Georgia Pappas

GEORGIA

Preschool Special Education
GA Department of Education
1970 Twin Towers East
Atlanta, GA 30334–5060
404/657–9955
Contact: Brenda Bachechi, Consultant

Local EI Program Support
Division of Public Health
Department of Human Resources
2 Peachtree Street, Room 7–315
Atlanta, GA 30303–3166
404/657–2726
Contact: Eve Bogan, Coordinator

Georgia Advocacy Office, Inc.
1708 Peachtree Street, NW Suite 505
Atlanta, GA 30309
404/885–1234
800/537–2329
Contact: Pat Powell, Exec Director

ARC of Georgia
2860 East Point Street, Suite 200
East Point, GA 30344
404/761–3150
Contact: Tom Query, Exec Director

University Affiliated Program of GA
for Persons with Developmental
Disabilities
University of Georgia
Dawson Hall
Athens, GA 30602
404/542–4827
Contact: Zolinda Stoneman, Exec Director

Parent to Parent of Georgia, Inc.
2939 Flowers Road, S.
Suite 131
Atlanta, GA 30341
404/451–5484
Contact: Kathleen Judd

Marcus Developmental Resource Center
at Emory University
1605 Chantilly Drive
Suite 100
Atlanta, GA 30324
404/727–9450
Contact: Peter Fanning, Ph.D.

Down Syndrome Association of Atlanta
1687 Tullie Circle, Suite 110
Atlanta, GA 30329
404/321–0877
Contact: Nancy Armstrong

Up With Downs
1329–A 18th Street
Columbus, GA 31901
404/327–5498
Contact: Anne Stumhofer

GUAM

Early Childhood Special Education
Department of Ed/Div of Special Education
PO Box DE
Agana, GU 96910
011/(671)646–8726
011/(671)646–1416
Contact: Faye E. Mata, Program Supervisor

Leilani T. Nishimura, Part H Coordinator
PO Box DE
Agana, GU 96910
011(671)475–0548

The Advocacy Office
PO Box 8830
Tamuning, GU 96911
011(671)646–9026
Contact: Eddie del Rosario, Director

Gaum Down Syndrome Association
30 Cruz Heights
Ipan, GU 96930
671/789-1208
Contact: Jessica Wilder

HAWAII

Special Education Section
HI Department of Education
3430 Leahi Avenue
Honolulu, HI 96815
808/737-3720
Contact: Margaret Donovan, Admin

Zero-to-3 Hawaii Project
Pan Am Bldg., 1600 Kapiolani Blvd., Suite
  1401
Honolulu, HI 96814
808/957-0066
Contact: Jean Johnson, Coordinator

Protection and Advocacy Agency
1580 Makaloa Street, Suite 1060
Honolulu, HI 96814
808/949-2922
Contact: Gary Smith, Exec Director

The Arc in Hawaii
3989 Diamond Head Road
Honolulu, HI 96816
808/737-7995
Contact: Ahmad Saidin, Exec Director

Hawaii University Affiliated Program
Developmental Disabilities, U of HI at
  Manoa
1776 University Avenue, UA 4-6
Honolulu, HI 96822
808/956-5009

Assisting with Appropriate Rights in Education (AWARE)
200 North Vineyard Blvd., #310
Honolulu, HI 96817
808/536-2280 (voice or TDD)
Contact: Edna Amuimuia, Project Coordinator

Special Parent Information Network
  (SPIN)
919 Ala Moana Blvd., #101
Honolulu, HI 96814
808/586-8126
Contact: Susan Rocco, Coordinator

Hawaii Down Syndrome Congress
419 Keoniana Street, Apt. 804
Honolulu, HI 96815
808/949-1999
Contact: Connie Smith

IDAHO

Special Education Section/ID Dept of
  Educ
PO Box 83720
Boise, ID 83720-0027
208/334-3940
Contact: Fred Balcom, Supervisor

Bureau of Developmental Disabilities
Dept of Health and Welfare
450 West State Street, 7th Floor
Boise, ID 83720-0036
208/334-5523
Contact: Mary Jones, Project Manager

Comprehensive Advocacy, Inc.
4477 Emerald Street, Suite B-100
Boise, ID 83706
208/336-5353
Contact: Shawn DeLoyola, Director

ID Center on Developmental Disabilities
University Affiliated Program/Univ of ID
129 W. Third Street
Moscow, ID 83843
208/885-6849
Contact: A. Lee Parks, Director

Idaho Parents Unlimited Inc. (IPUL)
4696 Overland Road, #478
Boise, ID 83705
800/242-4785
208/342-5884 (V/TDD)
Contact: Debra J. Johnson, Exec Director

Treasure Valley Down Syndrome Support
  Group
1411 E. Roosevelt
Nampa, ID 83686
208/465-5989
Contact: Dianna Brown

Down Syndrome Parents Support Group
1624 Sierra
Pocatello, ID 83201
208/237-7192
Contact: Shirley Ellsworth-Hawk

ILLINOIS

Department of Special Education
Illinois State Board of Education
100 North First Street, E233
Springfield, IL 62777–0001
217/782–6601
Contact: Pamela Reising, Sr. Consultant

Early Intervention Program
Illinois State Board of Education
100 West Randolph St., C-14–300
Chicago, IL 60601
312/814–5560
Contact: Audrey Witzman, Part H Coordinator

Protection and Advocacy, Inc.
11 East Adams, Suite 1200
Chicago, IL 60603
312/341–0022
Contact: Zena Naiditch, Director

The Arc of Illinois
925 West 175th Street, 3rd Floor
Homewood, IL 60430
708/206–1930
Contact: Anthony Paulauski, Exec Director

Univ Affiliated Program for Developmental Disabilities
1640 West Roosevelt Road
Chicago, IL 60608
312/413–1647
Contact: David Braddock, Director

Family Resource Center on Disabilities
20 East Jackson Blvd., Room 900
Chicago, IL 60604
312/939–3513
800/952–4194
312/939–3519 (TT)
Contact: Charlotte Des Jardins, Director

IL Alliance for Exceptional Children & Adults
8 Walton Place
Normal, IL 61761
309/452–9896 (V/TDD)
Contact: Charlene Trappe-Black, President

United Parent Support for Down Syndrome
550 Burnt Ember Lane
Buffalo Grove, IL 60089
708/520–5345

Contact: Bruce T. Marcus

Parent Association for Down Syndrome
Box 1180
Carbondale, IL 62901
618/549–4442
Contact: Tammy Beasley-Castellano

Caring Parents
825 18th Street, Box 587
Charleston, IL 61920–0587
217/348–0127
Contact: Sandra Boyer

Decatur Illinois Down Syndrome Association
2209 Grandview
Decatur, IL 62526
217/422–2056
Contact: Marshall Sperry

Avenues to Independence
1841 Busse Highway
Des Plaines, IL 60016
708/299–9720
Contact: Bob Okazaki

Elgin Area Down Syndrome Parent Support Group
Jane Shover Easter Seal
799 S. McLean Blvd.
Elgin, IL 60121
708/742–3264
Contact: Sandy Holm

Aurora Area Parents of Children with Down Syndrome
1309 Hill Road
Geneva, IL 60134
708/232–7485
Contact: Terri Brems

Down Syndrome Association of Champaign County
Box 797
Mahomet, IL 61853
217/586–4552
Contact: Vicki Niswander

Down Syndrome Association of Southwestern Illinois
Box 322
Glen Carbon, IL 62034

Central Illinois Down Syndrome Organization

Box 595
Normal, IL 61761
309/452–3264
Contact: Diane Crutcher

National Association for Down Syndrome
Box 4542
Oak Brook, IL 60522–4542
708/325–9112
Contact: Peggy Nemec

Down Syndrome Awareness
3216 Red Bud Lane
Springfield, IL 62707
217/529–8409
Contact: Edward & Elizabeth Brooks

Heart of Illinois Down Syndrome Association
PARC EIS
107 Siesta Drive
Washington, IL 61571
309/698–7778
Contact: Jackie Schwenk

INDIANA

Division of Special Education
State Department of Education
229 State House
Indianapolis, IN 46204
317/232–0570
Contact: Kathleen Hugo, Project Director

Div of Families & Children/Bur of Child
Development
402 West Washington Street, Room, W-386
Indianapolis, IN 46204
317/232–2429
Contact: Maureen Greer, Assistant Deputy Director

Indiana Advocacy Services
850 North Meridian Street, Suite 2–C
Indianapolis, IN 46204
317/232–1150
800/622–4845 (In IN)
Contact: Mary Lou Haynes, Exec Director

The Arc of Indiana
22 East Washington Street, Suite 210
Indianapolis, IN 46204
317/632–4387
Contact: John Dickerson, Exec Director

Institution for the Study of Dev Disabilities

Indiana University
2853 East Tenth Street
Bloomington, IN 47408–2601
812/855–9396 (TDD)
812/833–6508
Contact: Henry Schroeder, Director

Riley Child Development Center
Indiana University School of Medicine
James Whitcomb Riley Hospital for Children
702 Barnhill Drive, Room 5837
Indianapolis, IN 46202–5226
317/274–8167
Contact: John D. Rau, MD Director

IN*SOURCE
833 Northside Blvd., Bldg. #1 REAR
South Bend, IN 46617
219/234–7101
800/332–4433 (In IN)
Contact: Richard Burden, Exec Director

Indiana Parent Information Network, Inc.
4755 Kingway Drive, Ste 105
Indianapolis, IN 46205–1545
800/964–4746
317/257–8683
Contact: Donna Gore-Olsen, Exec Director

New Horizons Rehabilitation, Inc.
Box 98, 237 Six Pine
Ranch Road
Batesville, IN 47006
812/934–4528
Contact: Marie Dausch

DSA of Southeastern Indiana
418 Meadow Lane
Batesville, IN 47006
812/934–4697
Contact: Mary Freeland

Down Syndrome Support Association of
Central Indiana
10792 Downing Street
Carmel, IN 46032–3869
317/574–9757
Contact: Larry W. Kaser

Down Syndrome Association of NW Indiana, Inc.
2927 Jewett Avenue
Highland, IN 46322
219/838–3656
Contact: Anne Wadle

ROSEBUDS
1318 Elizabeth Street
Lafayette, IN 47904
317/742–8513
Contact: Kathi Mitchell

UPS FOR DOWNS
Box 385, 8322 Susan Court
Newburgh, IN 47629
812/853–7628
Contact: Sally Cash

Down Syndrome Family Support and Advocacy Group
Box 6579
South Bend, IN 46617
219/272–9591
Contact: Bonnie Hay

D.S. Support Association of South Indiana
3215 Chipaway Court
Floyds Knobs, IN 47119
812/923–5026
Contact: Ann Steiner

IOWA

Bureau of Special Educ/Dept of Educ
Grimes State Office Building
Des Moines, IA 50319–0146
515/281–3176
Contact: Joan Turner Clary, ECSE Consultant

Linda Gleissner, Part H Coordinator
133 Education Center
University of Northern Iowa
Cedar Falls, IA 50614
319/273–3299

Iowa Protection and Advocacy Services, Inc
3015 Merle Hay Road, Suite 6
Des Moines, IA 50310
515/278–2502
Contact: Mervin L. Roth, Director

The Arc of Iowa
715 East Locust
Des Moines, IA 50309
515/283–2358
Contact: Kit Olson, Exec Director

Iowa University Affiliated Program
Division of Developmental Disabilities
University Hospital School
The University of Iowa
Iowa City, IA 52242

319/353–6390
Contact: Alfred Healy, MD, Director

Iowa Pilot Parents, Inc.
33 North 12th Street
PO Box 1151
Fort Dodge, IA 50501
515/576–5870
800/952–4777
Contact: Kim Stuhrenberg, Acting Exec Director

Up with Downs Support Group
2301 Southridge Circle
Marshalltown, IA 50158
515/752–7075
Contact: Julie Lang

Siouxland Down Syndrome Support Group
PO Box 2171
Sioux City, IA 51104
712/276–3642
Contact: Robin Schomock

Up with Downs Family Support Group
8217 Sutton Drive
Urbandale, IA 50322
515/276–2544
Contact: Jan Mackey

KANSAS

Special Education Outcome
Kansas State Board of Education
120 East 10th Street
Topeka, KS 66612
913/296–3869
Contact: Betty Weithers, Team Leader

State Department of Health & Environment
Landon State Office Bldg.
900 SW Jackson, 10th Floor
Topeka, KS 66612–1290
913/296–6135
Contact: Marnie Campbell, Part H Coordinator

Kansas Advocacy & Protective Services
2601 Anderson Ave., Suite 200
Manhattan, KS 66502–2876
913/776–1541
800/432–8276
Contact: Joan Strickler, Exec Director

The Arc of Kansas
3601 SW 29th, Suite 237

Topeka, KS 66604
913/271–8783
Contact: Robert E. Geers, Coordinator

Kansas Univ Affiliated Program-Kansas City
Children's Rehab Univ/KS Univ Medical Center
3901 Rainbow Blvd
Kansas City, KS 66160–7340
913/588–5900
Contact: Donna Daily, MD Director

Kansas Univ Affiliated Facility-Lawrence
348 Haworth Hall/U of Kansas
Lawrence, KS 66045
913/864–4950
Contact: Steve Schroeder, Director

Prairie Pilot Parents
703 W. Second
Oakley, KS 67701
913/672–3125
Contact: Sharon Hixson

Down Syndrome Guild of Greater Kansas City, Inc.
8445 Linden Lane
Prairie Village, KS 66207
913/648–6464
Contact: June Rouse

Parent Support Group of Hays, KS
1315 285th Avenue
Hays, KS 67601
913/625–9700
Contact: Diane Steckline

Families Together
501 SW Jackson, Ste 400
Topeka, KS 66603
800/264–6343 (V/TYY) (in KS)
913/233–4777
Contact: Patricia Gerdel & Doug Gerdel

KENTUCKY

Office of Learning Program Development
Capitol Plaza Tower, 21st Floor
Frankfort, KY 40601
502/564–7056
Contact: Barbara Singleton, Preschool Consultant

Infant and Toddler Program, Dept of Mental Health &
Mental Retardation Services

275 East Main Street
Frankfort, KY 40621
502/564–7700
Contact: Jim Henson, Part H Coordinator

Dept for Public Advocacy, P&A Division
100 Fair Oaks Lane, Third Floor
Frankfort, KY 40601
502/564–2967
800/372–2988 (in KY) (Voice and TDD)
Contact: Gayla O. Peach, Director

The Arc of Kentucky
833 East Main
Frankfort, KY 40601
502/875–5225
Contact: Patty Dempsey, Asst Admin

Interdisciplinary Human Dev Institute
University Affiliated Facility
University of Kentucky
302 Mineral Industries Building
Lexington, KY 40506–0205
606/257–1714
Contact: Melton C. Martinson, Director

Kentucky Special Parent Involvement Network (KY-SPIN)
2210 Goldsmith Lane, Suite 118
Louisville, KY 40218
502/456–0923
800/525–7746
Contact: Paulette Logsdon, Director

Down Syndrome of Louisville
3713 Fallen Timber Drive
Louisville, KY 40241
502/339–8690
Contact: Gail Lowe

LOUISIANA

Preschool Programs, Office of Special Ed Services
Dept of Education
PO Box 94064
Baton Rouge, LA 70804–9064
504/342–3479
Contact: Janice K. Zube, Program Manager

Office of Special Education Services/Dept of Ed
PO Box 94064
Baton Rouge, LA 70804–9064
504/342–1837
Contact: Susan Batson, Admin, Preschool Programs

Advocacy Center for the Elderly & the Disabled
210 O'Keefe, Suite 700
New Orleans, LA 70112
504/522–2337
800/960–7705 (In LA)
Contact: Lois V. Simpson, Exec Director

The Arc of LA
PO Box 65129
Baton Rouge, LA 70896–5129
504/927–0764
Contact: Jim Brolin, Exec Director

Human Development Center
LA State University Medical Center
1100 Florida Avenue, Bldg #138
New Orleans, LA 70119
504/942–8200
Contact: Robert E. Crow, Director

Parent-to-Parent of LA Family Support
Program
200 Henry Clay Avenue
New Orleans, LA 70118
800/299–9511 (ext. 4268)
Contact: Peggy LeBlanc, Parent Coordinator

Down Syndrome Awareness Group
Box 15173
Baton Rouge, LA 70895
504/664–5171
Contact: Charmaine Neptune

Acadiana Down Syndrome Association
Box 32153
Lafayette, LA 70539
318/984–7488
Contact: Roy Brown

Southwest Down Syndrome Association
628 Cleveland Street
Lake Charles, LA 70601
318/433–2107
Contact: Donna Yancey

Up with Down's
450 Railsback Road
Shreveport, LA 71106
318/746–7643

DS Association of Greater New Orleans
PO Box 55204
Metairie, LA 70055–5204

504/889–8749
Contact: Bill Boustead

Southwest Louisiana DS Assoc
2314 17th Street
Lake Charles, LA 70601
318/477–5031
Contact: Nancy Authement

MAINE

Division of Special Education, Dept of Ed
State House, Station #23
Augusta, ME 04333–0023
207/289–5950
Contact: David Noble Stockford, Director

Child Development Services
State House, Station #146
Augusta, ME 04333
207/287–3272
Contact: Joanne C. Holmes, Part H and
Sect 619 Coordinator

Maine Advocacy Services
32 Winthrop Street, PO Box 2007
Augusta, ME 04338–2007
207/626–2774
800/452–1948 (in ME) (TDD)
Contact: Paul K. Vestal, Jr., Exec Director

Center for Community Inclusion, UAP
5703 Alumni Hall
University of Maine
Orono, ME 04469–5703
207/581–1084
Contact: Lucille A. Zeph, Director

Special Needs Parent Information Net-
work (SPIN)
PO Box 2067
Augusta, ME 04338–2067
207/582–2504
800/870–7746 (in ME)
Contact: Margaret Squires/Janice
LaChance

Maine Parent Federation
PO Box 2067
Augusta, ME 04338
800/870–7746 (V/TYY) (in ME)
207/582–2504

MARYLAND

Maryland Infants & Toddlers Program

One Market Center, Box 15
300 West Lexington Street, Suite 304
Baltimore, MD 21201
410/333-8100
Contact: Carol Ann Baglin, Director

Information & Referral Specialist
MD State Dept of Education
Division of Special Education
200 West Baltimore Street
Baltimore, MD 21201
410/333-2478
410/333-2666 (TDD)
Contact: Marjorie Shulbank

Maryland Disability Law Center
2510 St Paul Street
Baltimore, MD 21202
410/235-4700
Contact: Elizabeth Jones, Director

The Arc of Maryland
6810 Deerpath Road, Suite 310
Baltimore, MD 21227
410/379-0400
Contact: Cristine Boswell Marchand, Exec Director

Parents' Place of MD Inc.
7257 Parkway Drive, Suite 210
Hanover, MD 21076
410/712-0900
Contact: Larry Larsen, Director

Parent Support Network, Infants and Toddlers Program
One Market Center, Box 15
300 West Lexington, Suite 304
Baltimore, MD 21201
410/333-8100
Contact: Mona Freedman, Coordinator

Andrews Area PODS
6007 Clinton Way
Clinton, MD 20735
301/868-7673
Contact: Mary Alyce R. Bauer

Down Syndrome Parent Support Group of Washington County
Rt. 12, Box 80
Hagerstown, MD 21742
301/791-3587
Contact: Carol Alphin

FRIENDS
5612 Bartonsville Road

Frederick, MD 21701-6838
301/898-7628
Contact: Patti Saylor

Chesapeake Down Syndrome
Parent Group, Inc.
12103 Long Lake Dr.
Owings Mills, MD 21117
410/356-8496

Parents' Place of Western Maryland
23 E Frederick St.
Walkersville, MD 21793
800/735-2258 (V/TYY) (MD only)
301/898-0936

Montgomery County PODS
1160 Nebel Street
Rockville, MD 20852
301/984-5777
Contact: Joyce Glenner

MASSACHUSETTS

Early Learning Services
Department of Education
350 Main Street
Malden, MA 02148-5023
617/388-3300
Contact: Elisabeth Schaefer, Administrator

Early Intervention Services
Department of Public Health
150 Tremont Street, 7th Floor
Boston, MA 02111
617/727-5090
Contact: Andrea F. Schuman, Part H Coordinator

Disability Law Center, Inc.
11 Beacon Street, Suite 925
Boston, MA 02108
617/723-8455
Contact: Susan Herz, Exec Director

The Arc of Massachusetts
217 South Street
Waltham, MA 02154
617/891-6270
Contact: Leo Sarkissian, Exec Director

Developmental Evaluation Center
Children's Hospital
300 Longwood Avenue
Boston, MA 02115
617/735-6509

Contact: Allen C. Crocker, MD Director

Federation for Children with Special
Needs
95 Berkeley Street
Boston, MA 02116
617/482-2915
800/331-0688 (in MA)
Contact: Artie Higgins, Director

Greater Boston Association for Citizens
with Mental Retardantion and Related
Disabilities
1505 Commonwealth Avenue
Boston, MA 02135
617/783-3900
Contact: Kimberly Molle, Advocacy

Massachusetts Down Syndrome Congress
Box 866
Melrose, MA 02176
617/742-4440
Contact: Patricia Knipstein

Down Syndrome Mother's Group
78 Rounds Street
New Bedford, MA 02740
617/997-3975
Contact: Elaine Holland

Mental Health Association of Greater
Springfield
146 Chestnut Street
Suite 400
Springfield, MA 01103
413/734-2376

MICHIGAN

Comprehensive Program in Health &
Early Childhood
Department of Education
PO Box 30008
Lansing, MI 48909
517/373-2537
Contact: Jacquelyn Thompson, Consultant

Michigan Protection and Advocacy Service
106 West Allegan, Suite 210
Lansing, MI 48933-1706
517/487-1755
Contact: Elizabeth W. Bauer, Exec Director

The Arc MI

313 South Washington, Suite 200
Lansing, MI 48933
517/487-5426
Contact: Marjorie Mitchell, Exec Director

Developmental Disabilities Institute
Wayne State University
326 Justice Building
6001 Cass Avenue
Detroit, MI 48202
313/577-2654, 2655
Contact: Michael Peterson, Director

Citizens Alliance to Uphold Special Education (CAUSE)
313 South Washington Square, Suite 040
Lansing, WI 48933
517/485-4084
800/221-9105 (in MI)
Contact: Sue Pratt, Exec Director

Parents Training Parents Project
23077 Greenfield Road, Suite 205
Southfield, MI 48075-3745
810/557-5070
Contact: Martha Wilson, Project Coordinator

Family Support Network
1200 6th St., 9th Floor
Detroit, MI 48226
313/256-3682
800/359-3722

Washtenaw Down Syndrome Support
Group
2624 Essex Road
Ann Arbor, MI 48104
313/971-3124
Contact: Barbara Conlon

University of Michigan Hospitals Pediatric
Genetics
D1109 Medical Pro. Bldg.
Box 0718
Ann Arbor, MI 48109-0718
313/764-0579

Down Syndrome Association of Livingston
County
7485 Herbst Road
Brighton, MI 48116
313/229-6196
313/227-7219
Contact: Laurie Beltowski

Down Syndrome Support Group St. Clair
County
2509 Woodstock Dr
Port Huron, MI 48060
810/987–5481
Contact: Helen Kivel

Down Syndrome Resource League
2621 Lorraine Avenue
Kalamazoo, MI 49008
616/345–0690
Contact: Ron Denardo

Down Syndrome Association of West
Michigan
Box 8804
Kentwood, MI 49518
616/956–3488
Contact: Peg Fakler

Down Syndrome Association of Marquette
Alger
427 W. College Avenue
Marquette, MI 49855
906/228–9400
Contact: Sylvia Carter

Family Focus on Down Syndrome
828 Ten Point Drive
Rochester Hills, MI 48309
313/652–4073
Contact: Elizabeth Monroe

Never Say Never
2235 Delaware Blvd
Saginaw, MI 48602
517/799–8654
Contact: Trish or Joe Bronz

Families Exploring Down Syndrome
Box 982
Sterling Heights, MI 48311–0982
313/977–3259
Contact: William A. Brown

Down Syndrome Association of Northwest
Michigan
Box 1451
Traverse City, MI 49684
616/922–4922
Contact: Christopher Keister

Parents of Children with Down Syndrome,
Inc.
1603 N. Pleasant
Royal Oak, MI 48067
313/827–9135

810/855–3968
Contact: Barb Malasky

Parents/Friends of Down Syndrome Children
4265 Halkirk
Waterford, MI 48095
313/623–9660
Contact: Lawrence Hearn

MINNESOTA

Community Collaboration Team, Dept of
Educ
Capitol Square Bldg., Room 827
550 Cedar Street
St. Paul, MN 55101
612/296–5007
Contact: Robyn Widley, ECSE Specialist

Interagency Early Intervention Project
for Young Children with Disabilities and
Their Families
Department of Education
Capitol Square Bldg., Room 927
550 Cedar Street
St. Paul, MN 55101
612/296–7032
Contact: Jan Rubeinstein, Part H Coordi-
nator

Minnesota Disability Law Center
430 First Avenue, N Suite 300
Minneapolis, MN 55401–1780
612/332–1441
Contact: Luther Granquist, Managing Attorney

Institute on Community Integration
(UAP)
University of Minnesota
102 Pattee Hall
Minneapolis, MN 55455
612/624–6300
Contact: Scott McConnell, Director

PACER Center, Inc.
4826 Chicago Avenue South
Minneapolis, MN 55417–1098
612/827–2966
800/53–PACER (in MN)
Contact: Marge & Paula F. Goldberg

Down Syndrome Association of Minnesota
PO Box 22626
Minneapolis, MN 55422

612/339–5544
Contact: Susan Gill

Pilot Parents
201 Ordean Bldg.
Duluth, MN 55802
218/726–4725
Contact: Addie Jessenein

St. Cloud Down Syndrome Support Group
Box 1536
St. Cloud, MN 56302
612/251–0666
Contact: Marie Kilgin

MISSISSIPPI

Bureau of Special Services
Department of Education
PO Box 771
Jackson, MI 39205–0771
601/359–3498
Contact: Nancy Artigues, Coordinator

Infant & Toddler Program
MS State Dept of Health (MSDH)
PO Box 1700
2423 North State Street, Room 105A
Jackson, MS 39215–1700
601/960–7622
800/451–3903
Contact: Hope Bacon, Part H Coordinator

MS P&A System for DD Inc.
5330 Executive Place, Suite A
Jackson, MS 39206
601/981–8207
Contact: Rebecca Floyd, Exec Director

MS University Affiliated Program
University of Southern Mississippi
Southern Station, Box 5163
Hattiesburg, MS 39406–5163
601/266–5163
Contact: Jane Z. Siders, Director

Parent Partners
ARC of Mississippi
3111 N. State Street
Jackson, MS 39216
601/366–5707
800/366–5707 (in MS)
Contact: Lynn Armstrong, Director

Mississippi Parent Network
PO Box 5895
Pearl, MS 39209

601/932–1116
Contact: Kathy Odle-Pounds, Director

DS Association of Corinth
Alcorn County Courthouse
Corinth, MS 38834
601/287–4649
Contact: Mike Wamsley

Down's Parents of Jackson
PO Box 12598
Jackson, MS 39236–2598
601/366–1004
Contact: Tammy Thomas

MISSOURI

Coordinator of Special Education
Department of Elementary and Secondary
Education
PO Box 480
Jefferson City, MO 65102
314/751–4909
Contact: John Heskett

Department of Early Childhood Special
Education
Department of Elementary and Secondary
Education
PO Box 480
Jefferson City, MO 65102
314/751–0185
Contact: Melodie Friedebach, ECSE Director

MO Protection & Advocacy Service
925 South Country Club Drive, Unit B-1
Jefferson City, MO 65109
314/893–3333
800/392–8667 (in MO)
Contact: Cynthia N. Schloss, PhD Director

Univ Affiliated Program for Developmental Disabilities
University of MO at Kansas City
Institute for Human Development
2220 Holmes Street
Kansas City, MO 64108
816/235–1770
Contact: Carl F. Calkins, Director

Missouri Parents Act-IMPACT
1722W South Glenstone, Suite 125
Springfield, MO 65804
417/882–7434
800/743–7634 (in MO)
Contact: Marianne Toombs, Exec Director

Missouri Parents Act-IMPACT
8631 Delmar, Suite 300
St. Louis, MO 63124
314/997–7622
800/995–3160
Contact: Beth Mollenkamp, Program Coordinator

Missouri Parents Act-IMPACT
3100 Main St., Suite 303
Kansas City, MO 64111
816/531–7070
Contact: Carolyn Stewart, Program Director

Down Syndrome Association of Mid-Missouri
5123 Mont Street
Columbia, MO 65203
314/443–7831
Contact: Diane & Rik Barker

Mineral Area Down Syndrome Organization
538 Sherwood Lane
Farmington, MO 63640
314/756–5424
Contact: John Bird

Down Syndrome Guild of Greater Kansas City, Inc.
636 W. 57th Terrace
Kansas City, MO 64113
816/444–2755
Contact: Shelley Stander

Down Syndrome Association of St. Louis, Inc.
7269 Dartmouth
St. Louis, MO 63130
314/725–6371
Contact: Mary Hart

MONTANA

Division of Special Education/Office of Public Instruction
State Capitol
Helena, MT 59620
406/444–4425
Contact: Dan McCarthy, Preschool Specialist

Developmental Disabilities Division
Dept of Social & Rehabilitation Services
PO Box 4210
Helena, MT 56904

406/444–2995
Contact: Jan Spiegle, Part H Coordinator

Montana Advocacy Program
PO Box 1680, 316 North Park, Room 211
Helena, MT 56924
406/444–3889
800/245–4743 (in MT)
Contact: Kris Bakula, Exec Director

Montana Univ Affiliated Rural Inst on Disabilities
52 Corbin Hall
The University of Montana
Missoula, MT 59812
406/243–5467
800/732–0323
Contact: Tom Seekins, Acting Director

Parents Let's Unite for Kids (PLUK)
EMC/Special Educ Bldg., Room 267
1500 North 30th Street
Billings, MT 59101–0298
406/657–2055
Contact: Kathy Kelker, Director

NEBRASKA

Special Education Section
State Dept of Education
PO Box 94987
Lincoln, NE 68509
402/471–2471
Contact: Judy Constantin, Coordinator

Nebraska Advocacy Services, Inc.
522 Lincoln Center Bldg., 215 Centennial Mall South
Lincoln, NE 68508
402/474–3183
800/422–6691
Contact: Timothy Shaw, Exec Director

The Arc of Nebraska
521 South 14th Street, Suite 211
Lincoln, NE 68508
402/475–4407
Contact: Ginger Clubine, Exec Director

Meyer Rehabilitation Institute
University of Nebraska Medical Center
600 South 42nd Street
Omaha, NE 68198–5450
402/559–6430
Contact: Bruce A. Buehler, MD Director

Nebraska Parent's Information & Training Center
3610 Dodge Street, Suite 102
Omaha, NE 68131
402/346–0525 (V/TT)
800/284–8520 (V/TT in NE)
Contact: Jean Sigler, Project Director

Pilot Parents
3610 Dodge Street
Omaha, NE 68110
402/346–5220
Contact: Annie Adamson, Coordinator

Pilot Parents Program
410 Lincoln Center Bldg.
215 Centennial Mall, S.
Suite 410
Lincoln, NE 68508
402/477–6925
Contact: Donna Bolz

NEVADA

Special Education Branch, Dept of Education
400 West King Street, Capitol Complex
Carson City, NV 89710
702/687–3140
Contact: Sharon Rogers, Coordinator

Early Childhood Services/DCFS
Department of Human Resources
3987 S. McCarren Blvd.
Reno, NV 89502
702/688–2284
Contact: Marilyn K. Walter, Chief

Office of Protection and Advocacy
1135 Terminal Way, Suite 105
Reno, NV 89502
702/688–1233
800/992–5715 (in NV)
Contact: Travis Wall, Director

NV Parent Connection
3380 S. Arville Blvd, Suite J
Las Vegas, NV 89102
702/252–0259 (ext 112)
800/508–4464
Contact: Barbara Bernabei, Director

NV Parent Connection
Carson City, NV
800/289–3495
Contact: Cindy Pennington

Southern Nevada Down Syndrome Organization
3601 W. Sahara Avenue
Suite 203
Las Vegas, NV 89102
702/222–1970
Contact: Lauren Cobey

NEW HAMPSHIRE

Special Education Bureau, Dept of Education
State Office Park, South
101 Pleasant Street
Concord, NH 03301–3860
603/271–3741
Contact: Ruth Littlefield, Program Coordinator

NH Infants and Toddlers Program
Division of Mental Health & Dev Services
Hospital Administration Bldg.
105 Pleasant Street
Concord, NH 03301–3860
603/271–5122
Contact: Donna Schlachman, Part H Coordinator

Disabilities Rights Center, Inc.
PO Box 19
Concord, NH 03302–0019
603/228–0432
Contact: Donna Woodfin, Exec Director

The Arc of NH
10 Ferry Street, Box 4
The Concord Center
Concord, NH 03301
603/228–9092
Contact: Paula Bundy

Parent Information Center (PIC)
PO Box 1422
Concord, NH 03302–1422
603/224–7005
603/224–6299
Contact: Judith Raskin, Director

Northern New England Down Syndrome Congress
PO Box 2314
Concord, NH 03302
603/938–2655
Contact: Michelle Zick

NEW JERSEY

Office of Special Education Program, Dept of Education
225 West State Street, CN 500
Trenton, NJ 08625
609/633–6833
Contact: Jeffrey Osowski, Director

Division of Special Education/Dept of Education
225 West State Street, CN 500
Trenton, NJ 08625
609/292–7604
Contact: Arlene Roth, Manager Early Childhood Education

Division of Advocacy for the Developmentally Disabled
Department of the Public Advocate
CN850, Trenton, NJ 08625
609/292–9742
609/633–7106 (TTY)
800/922–7233 (in NJ)
Contact: Sarah W. Mitchell, Director

The Arc of NJ
985 Livingston Avenue
North Brunswick, NJ 08902
201/246–2525
Contact: Paul Potito, Exec Director

The University Affiliated Program of NJ
UMDNJ, New Jersey's U of the Health Sciences
Robert Wood Johnson Medical School, Brookwood II
45 Knightsbridge Road
PO Box 6810
Piscataway, NJ 08855–6810
908/463–4407 (TDD)
908/463–4447
Contact: Deborah Spitalnik, PhD, Exec Director

Statewide Parent Advocacy Network (SPAN)
516 North Avenue, East
Westfield, NJ 07090
908/654–7726
800/654–7726
Contact: Diana Cuthbertson, Exec Director

"21 Downs"
PO Box 456

Cape May Court House, NJ 08210
609/263–5143
Contact: Jeanie Larsen

American Self-Help Clearinghouse
St. Clares-Riverside Medical Center
Denville, NJ 07834
800/367–6274
201/625–7101

Down Syndrome Support Group of South Jersey, Inc.
401 4th Avenue
Haddon Heights, NJ 08035
609/547–6773
Contact: Joanne McKeown

New Jersey Coalition for Down Syndrome
5 Union Hill Lane
Hazlet, NJ 07730
908/264–0824
Contact: Joan Bace

Down Syndrome Parent to Parent
Arc of Essex
7 Regent Street
Livingston, NJ 07039
201/535–1181
Contact: Lee Bergman

Down Syndrome Association of Central New Jersey
7 Fieldston Road
Princeton, NJ 08540
609/452–9139
908/747–5310
Contact: Joan Nester

Down Syndrome Parent Support Group
35 Haddon Avenue
Shrewsbury, NJ 07702
908/747–5310
Contact: Susan Levine

Down Syndrome Congress of Northern New Jersey
PO Box 43164
Upper Montclair, NJ 07043
201/744–3617
Contact: Joan Smith & Carmela Bal

Keeping Involved with Down Syndrome
PO Box 2301
Vineland, NJ 08360
609/696–1643
Contact: Lisa Willis

NEW MEXICO

Special Education Unit, Dept of Education
300 Don Gaspar Avenue
Santa Fe, NM 87501–2786
505/827–6541
Contact: Diane Turner, Coordinator

Department of Health
Development Disabilities Division
1190 St. Francis Drive
PO Box 26110
Santa Fe, NM 87502–6110
505/827–2573
Contact: Marilyn Price, Part H Coordinator

Protection and Advocacy System, Inc.
1720 Louisiana Blvd., NE Suite 204
Albuquerque, NM 87110
505/256–3100
800/432–4682 (in NM)
Contact: James Jackson, Exec Director

The Arc of NM
3500–G Comanche, NE
Albuquerque, NM 87107
505/883–4630
505/883–4630
Contact: John Foley, Exec Director

Project Adobe, Parents Reaching Out
(PRO)
1127 University Blvd., NE
Albuquerque, NM 87102
505/842–9045
800/524–5176 (in NM)
Contact: Sallie Van Curen, Exec Director

STEP*HI Parent/Infant Program
New Mexico School for the Deaf
1060 Cerrillos Road
Santa Fe, NM 87501
505/827–6789 (V/TDD)
Contact: Rosemary Gallegos, Coordinator

Education for Parent of Indian Children
with Special Needs/(EPICS) Project
PO Box 788
Bernalillo, NM 87004
505/867–3396
800/765–7320 (V/TDD)

Down Syndrome Association of
Albuquerque
4101 Central Avenue NW
Suite L-119

Albuquerque, NM 87105
505/831–5464
Contact: Deb Garcia

Parents Reaching Out to Help
870 Navajo Lane
Rio Rancho, NM 87124
505/891–2409
Contact: Cathie Thomas

NEW YORK

State Education Department
Special Education Dept.
1 Commerce Plaza, Educ Bldg., Room 1610
Albany, NY 12234
518/474–5548
Contact: Sandra Rybaltowski

Early Intervention Program
Bureau of Children and Adolescent Health
Corning Tower, Room 208
Albany, NY 12237
518/473–7016
Contact: Frank Zollo, Director

NY Comm on Quality of Care for the Mentally Disabled
99 Washington Avenue, Suite 1002
Albany, NY 12210
518/473–7378
Contact: Marcel Chaine, Advocacy Bureau

NYSARC, Inc.
393 Delaware Avenue
Delmar, NY 12054
518/439–8311

DD Center/St. Lukes-Roosevelt Hospital
Center
College of Physicians & Surgeons-Colum-
bia Univ
428 West 59th Street
New York, NY 10019
212/523–6230
Contact: Madeline W. Appell, Director

WIHD/University Affiliated Program
Westchester County Medical Center
Valhalla, NY 10595
914/285–8204
Contact: Ansley Bacon, Director

Parent Network Center
1443 Main Street
Buffalo, NY 14209
716/885–1004

800/724–7408 (in NY)
Contact: Joan M. Watkins, Director

Advocates for Children of New York (NY City)
24–16 Bridge Plaza South
Long Island, NY 11101
718/729–8866
Contact: Elizabeth C. Yeampierre

Family Support Project for the DD
North Central Bronx Hospital
3424 Kossuth Avenue, Room 15A10
Bronx, NY 10467
717/519–4796
717/519–4797
Contact: Mary Bonsignore, Project Coordinator

Down Syndrome/Aim High, Inc.
Box 12–624
Albany, NY 12212
518/381–9733
Contact: Joanne Fitzgerald

Down Syndrome Parent Support Group of Genessee County, Inc.
3770 Pike Road
Batavia, NY 14020
716/344–2092
Contact: Kay Cook

Association for Children with Down Syndrome
2616 Martin Avenue
Bellmore, NY 11710
516/221–4700
Contact: Fredda Stimell

Down Syndrome Association of St. Lawrence County
Star Route, PO Box 172
Canton, NY 13617
315/386–2018
Contact: Jackie Sauter

Down Syndrome Parent Group of Long Island
Box 287
East Setauket, NY 11733–0287
516/696–0564
Contact: Lisa Campbell

Down Syndrome Parent Group of Western New York, Inc.
547 Englewood Avenue
Kenmore, NY 14223

716/832–9334
Contact: Carol Hetzelt

Down Syndrome Support Group of Cattaraugus County
Box 1015
Olean, NY 14760
716/373–3026
Contact: Julie A. Stavish

Down Syndrome Parents Group of Queens
Box 81
Ozone Park, NY 11417
718/848–2548
Contact: Linda Glazebrook

Parent Assistance Committee on Down Syndrome
208 Lafayette Avenue
Peekskill, NY 10566
914/739–4085
Contact: Barbara Levitz

Flower City Down Syndrome Network
80 Karlan Drive
Rochester, NY 14617
716/338–2101
Contact: Laura Khedarian

Mid-Hudson Valley Down Syndrome Congress, Inc.
14 Zerner Blvd.
Hopewell Junction, NY 12533–9804
914/658–8419
Contact: David Wurtz

Down Syndrome Adoption Exchange
56 Midchester Avenue
White Plains, NY 10606
914/428–1236

DS Association of Central NY
PO Box 5
Manlius, NY 13104–0005
315/637–9711
315/682–4289
Contact: Shari Bottego

NORTH CAROLINA

Exceptional Children Support Team
Department of Public Instruction
301 N. Wilmington St., Educ Bldg., #570
Raleigh, NC 27601–2825
919/715–1565
Contact: E. Lowell Harris, Director

MH, DD & Substance Abuse Services
Department of Human Resources
325 North Salisbury Street
Raleigh, NC 27603
919/733-3654
Contact: Duncan Munn, Branch Head of
Day Services

Governor's Advocacy Council for Persons
with Disabilities
1318 Dale Street, Suite 100
Raleigh, NC 27605
919/733-9250
Contact: Cindy Crouse-Martin, Director

The Arc of North Carolina
16 Rowan Street, PO Box 20545
Raleigh, NC 27619
919/782-4632
Contact: Dave Richard, Exec Director

Clinical Center for the Study of Develop-
ment and Learning
CB# 7255, BSRC
University of North Carolina
Chapel Hill, NC 27599-7255
919/966-5171
Contact: Melvin Levine, MD Director

ECAC, Inc. (Exceptional Children's Assistance Center)
PO Box 16
Davidson, NC 28036
704/892-1321
800/962-6817 (in NC)
Contact: Connie Hawkins, Director

Family Support Network
CB #7340
University of NC at Chapel Hill
Chapel Hill, NC 27599-7340
919/966-2841
800/852-0042

Down Syndrome Association of Charlotte,
Inc.
Box 3136
Charlotte, NC 28210
704/536-2163
Contact: Toni Robinson

Supportworks: The Self-Help Clearinghouse
1012 Kings Drive
Suite 923
Charlotte, NC 28283

704/331-9500
Contact: Joal Fischer, MD

Piedmont Down Syndrome Support Network
202 Sonata Drive
Lewisville, NC 27203
919/945-3803
Contact: Carolyn Myracle

B.A.B.I.E.S.
650 N. Highland Avenue
Winston-Salem, NC 27101
919/725-7527
Contact: Chris Kelsey

PARENTS Project
300 Enola Road
Morganton, NC 28655
704/433-2662

NORTH DAKOTA

Special Education Div., Dept of Public In-
struction
State Capitol
Bismarck, ND 58505-6440
701/224-2277
Contact: Allan Ekblad, Coordinator

Development Disabilities Division
Department of Human Services
State Capitol, 600 East Boulevard Avenue
Bismarck, ND 58505-0270
701/224-2768
Contact: Robert Graham, Part H Coordina-
tor

Protection & Advocacy Project
400 East Broadway, Suite 515
Bismarck, ND 58501
702/244-2972
800/472-2670 (in ND)
Contact: Barbara C. Braun, Director

The Arc of North Dakota
418 East Rosser
PO Box 2776
Bismarck, ND 58502-2776
701/223-5349

Pathfinder Family Center
16th Street and 2nd Avenue, SW
Arrowhead Shopping Center
Minot, ND 58701
701/852-9426
701/852-9436

800/245–5840 (in ND)
Contact: Kathryn Erickson, Director

Down Syndrome Parent Support Group
2500 DeMers Avenue
Grand Forks, ND 58201
701/772–9191
Contact: Dianne Sheppard

OHIO

Div of Special Education
State Dept of Education
933 High Street
Worthington, OH 43085–4017
614/466–2650
Contact: John Herner, Director

Division of Early Childhood
State Dept of Education
65 South Front Street, Room 309
Columbus, OH 43266–0308
614/466–0224
Contact: Jane Wiechel, Director

Ohio Legal Rights Service
8 East Long Street, 5th Floor
Columbus, OH 43215
614/466–7264
800/282–9181 (in OH)
Contact: Carolyn Knight, Exec Director

The Arc of Ohio
1335 Dublin Road, Suite 205–C
Columbus, OH 43215
614/487–4720
800/875–2723
Contact: Ray Ferguson, Exec Director

Univ Affiliated Cincinnati Center for De-
velopmental Disorders
Pavillion Bldg., Elland & Bethesda Avenues
Cincinnati, OH 45229
513/589–4623
Contact: Jack H. Rubenstein, MD Director

UAP The Nisonger Center
321 McCampbell Hall, 1581 Dodd Drive
Columbus, OH 43210–1296
614/292–8365
Contact: Steven Reiss, Director

Child Advocacy Center
1821 Summit Rd #303
Cincinnati, OH 45237
513/821–2400 (V/TTY)

Contact: Cathy Keizman, Exec Director

OH Coalition for the Educ of Handicapped Children
1299 Campbell Road
Marion, OH 43302
800/374–2806
Contact: Martha Music, Parent Assistance

Northeast Ohio Down Syndrome Organiza-
tion
Box 4420
Austintown, OH 44515
216/792–0329
Contact: Holly Myers

United Parent Support for Down Syndrome
618 Second Street, NW
Suite 10
Canton, OH 44703
216/453–2727
Contact: Carol Lichtenwalter

Down Syndrome Association of Greater
Cincinnati
1821 Summit Road
Suite 102
Cincinnati, OH 45237
513/761–5400
Contact: Mary Grover/Jane Page-Sneider

Baker International Resource Ctr for
Down Syndrome
2800 Euclid Avenue
Suite 200
Cleveland, OH 44115
216/621–5858
800/899–3039
Contact: Florence Mitchell

Down Syndrome Association of Central
Ohio
933 High Street
Suite 106–A
Worthington, OH 43085
614/292–6297
Contact: Sherrie Andrus

Ohio Down Syndrome Organization
933 High Street
Suite 106–A
Worthington, OH 43085
614/431–2060
Contact: Brad Lynn

Miami Valley Down Syndrome Association

1444 Beaver Creek Lane
Kettering, OH 45429–3704
513/294–1240
Contact: Patti Ann Dixon

Down Syndrome Association of North Central Ohio
43 Darby Drive
Lexington, OH 44904
419/884–0605
Contact: Anita Miller

St. Rita's Down Syndrome Parent Group
730 West Market Street
Lima, OH 45801
419/226–9019
Contact: Jane D. Schmidt

First Down
8720 Bechtel Rd.
Elyria, OH 44035
440/323-0724
Contact: Lori Govich

UpSide of Downs of Greater Cleveland
8251 Winthrop Court
Mentor, OH 44060
216/255–8942
Contact: Paula Patterson

Down Syndrome Association of Greater Toledo
Box 502
Toledo, OH 43693
419/666–0233
Contact: Terry Perry

OKLAHOMA

Special Education Section, Dept of Education
2500 North Lincoln Blvd., Room 411
Oklahoma City, OK 73105
405/521–4876
Contact: Jill Burroughs, Asst Director

Special Education Section, Dept of Education
2500 North Lincoln Blvd., Room 411
Oklahoma City, OK 73105–4599
405/521–4880
Contact: Cathy Perri, Early Intervention Administrator

OK Disability Law Center, Inc.
4150 South 100th East Avenue
210 Cherokee Bldg.

Tulsa, OK 74146
918/664–5883 (V/TT)
800/226–5883 (V/TT in OK)
Contact: Steven A. Novick, Exec Director

Parents Reaching Out in OK (PRO-Oklahoma)
1917 South Harvard Avenue
Oklahoma City, OK 73128
405/681–9710
800/PL94–142 (V/TDD)
Contact: Sharon Bishop, Director

Parents of Children with Down Syndrome
4510 Beckett Court
Norman, OK 73072
405/321–4706
Contact: Jan Watts

Down Syndrome Association of Tulsa, Inc.
Box 54877
Tulsa, OK 74155
918/455–1475
Contact: Anita Montgomery

Parents of Children with Down Syndrome
132 Pinewood
Tuttle, OK 73089
405/381–2778
Contact: Sharon Richardson

OREGON

Division of Special Education, Dept of Education
700 Pringle Parkway, SE
Salem, OR 97310
503/378–3598
Contact: Sandi Fink, Coordinator

Early Intervention Programs
Mental Health Division
Department of Education
700 Pringle Parkway, SE
Salem, OR 97301
503/378–3598
Contact: Diane Allen, Coordinator

Oregon Advocacy Center
625 Board of Trade Bldg.
Portland, OR 97204–2309
503/243–2081
Contact: Robert Joondeph, Exec Director

The Arc of Oregon
1745 State Street
Salem, OR 97301

503/581-2726

Center on Human Development
Clinical Services Bldg.
University of OR-Eugene
Eugene, OR 97403
503/686-3591
Contact: Hill M. Walker, Director

Child Development & Rehabilitation Center
OR Health Sciences University
PO Box 574
Portland, OR 97207
503/494-8364
Contact: Gerald M. Smith, Director

Oregon COPE Project
(Coalition in OR for Parent Education)
999 Locust Street, NE
Salem, OR 97303
503/373-7477 (Voice/TDD)
Contact: Cheron Mayhall, Director

Pilot Parent Program
ARC Multnomah County
619 SW 11th Avenue
Suite 234
Portland, OR 97205-2692
503/223-7279
Contact: Lisa Adams-Reese

Down Syndrome Support Group
2731 SW Taylors Ferry Road
Portland, OR 97219
503/244-5128
Contact: Joan Medlen

PENNSYLVANIA

Bureau of Special Education
Department of Education
333 Market Street
Harrisburg, PA 17126-0333
717/783-6913
Contact: Rick Price, Special Education Advisor

Division of Early Intervention Services
Office of Mental Retardation
PO Box 2675
Harrisburg, PA 17105-2675
717/783-4873
Contact: Jacqueline Epstein, Part H
Coordinator

PA Protection & Advocacy, Inc.

116 Pine Street
Harrisburg, PA 17101
717/236-8110
800/692-7443 (in PA)
Contact: Kevin Casey, Exec Director

The Arc of Pennsylvania
123 Foster Street
Harrisburg, PA 17102
717/234-2621
Contact: W.A. West, Exec Director

Institute on Disabilities
Temple University, Ritter Annex 423
(004-00)
Philadelphia, PA 19122
215/204-1356 (V/TT)
Contact: Diane Nelson Bryen, PhD

Parent Education Network
333 East 7th Avenue
York, PA 17404
717/845-9722
800/522-5827 (V/TDD) (in PA)
800/441-5028 (Spanish)
Contact: Louise Thieme, Director

Down Syndrome Group of Western Pennsylvania, Inc.
923 McLaughlin Run Road
Bridgeville, PA 15017
412/221-1372
Contact: Lori Sanker

Down Syndrome Parent Group
927 West 22nd Street
Erie, PA 16502
814/455-9621
Contact: Rhonda Schember

Down Syndrome Interest Group
540 Cowpath Road
Hatfield, PA 19440
215/362-6375
Contact: Laura Heckler

Down Syndrome Today, Inc.
481 Baker Road
Freedom, PA 15042
412/728-2896
Contact: Linda Uhernik

Down Syndrome Support Group of
Lancaster County
93 Urban Drive
Lancaster, PA 17603
717/397-5023

Contact: Sharon K. Bertz

Down Syndrome Center of Western Pennsylvania
Childrens Hospital
1 Childrens Place
Pittsburgh, PA 15213
412/692–5560
Contact: William I. Cohen, MD

Parents of Down Syndrome, Inc.
Rt. 2 Box 497
Slatington, PA 18080
215/767–7736
Contact: Sheila Stasko

Delaware County Down Syndrome
Box 226
Springfield, PA 19064
215/896–7519
Contact: Paul Thomas

Pocono Parents of Down Syndrome
7136 Long Woods Road
Tobyhanna, PA 18466
717/894–0946
Contact: Diane Siani

Down Syndrome Interest Group-Chester
County
c/o ARC-Chester County
23 S New Street
West Chester, PA 19382
215/436–6740
Contact: Holly Healy

Up Side of Downs
412 Highland Avenue
Clarks Summit, PA 18411
717/586–7233
Contact: Dolores T. Waters

Down Syndrome Support Group of Berks
County
4800 6th Avenue
Temple, PA 19560
215/372–9053
215/929–8189
Contact: Barb Casse or Noe

Down Syndrome Support Group of Berks
County
845 N. 3rd Street
Reading, PA 19601–2505
215/929–8189
Contact: Barb Casse

PUERTO RICO

Assistant Secretary of Special Education
Department of Education
PO Box 190759
Hato Rey, PR 00919–0759
809/759–7228
Contact: Dr. Adela Vazquez Costa

Infants & Toddlers Program
Department of Health
Call Box 70184
San Juan, PR 00936
809/767–0870 Ext 2228
Contact: Carmen Aviles, Coordinator

Office of the Ombudsman for People with
Disabilities
PO Box 4234
San Juan, PR 00919
809/766–2388
Contact: David Cruz Belez, Ombudsman

Asociacion De Padres Pro Bienestar
Ninos Impedidos de PR, Inc.
Box 21301
San Juan, PR 00928–1301
809/763–4665
809/763–0345
809/250–4552 (TT)
Contact: Carmen Selles Vila, Project Director

Puerto Rico Down Syndrome Foundation
Box 1621
Dorado, PR 00646
809/796–2698
Contact: Miriam P. Perez de Martinez

RHODE ISLAND

Preschool ECSE Consultant
Special Education Program Services Unit
Dept of Elementary & Secondary Education
Roger Williams Bldg., Rm 209
22 Hayes Street
Providence, RI 02908
401/277–2705
Contact: Amy Cohen

Division of Family Health
State Department of Health
3 Capital Hill, Rm 302
Providence, RI 02908–5097

401/277–2313
401/277–2312
Contact: Ron Caladrone, Part H Coordinator

Rhode Island P&A System, Inc (RIPAS)
151 Broadway
Providence, RI 02903
401/831–3150
401/831–5335 (TDD)
Contact: Raymond L. Bandusky, Exec Director

Rhode Island Arc
99 Bald Hill Road
Cranston, RI 02920
401/463–9191
Contact: James Healey, Exec Director

Child Development Center, Rhode Island Hospital
593 Eddy Street
Providence, RI 02902
401/277–5681
Contact: Siegfried Pueschel, MD, Director

RI Parent Info Network (RIPIN)
500 Prospect Street
Pawtucket, RI 02860
401/727–4151
800/464–3399 (in RI)
Contact: Deenna Forist, Exec Director

Down Syndrome Society of Rhode Island
99 Bald Hill Road
Cranston, RI 02920
401/463–5751
Contact: Roberta Wexler

SOUTH CAROLINA

Office of Programs for Exceptional Children
1429 Senate Street, Fifth Floor, Room 511
Columbia, SC 29201
803/734–8126
Contact: Mary Ginn, Education Associate

Division of Rehab Services/Baby Net
Robert Mills Complex, Box 101106
Columbia, SC 29201
803/737–4046
Contact: Kathy Purnell, Interim Part H Coord.

SC P&A System for the Handicapped, Inc.
3710 Landmark Drive, Suite 208

Columbia, SC 29204
803/782–0639
800/922–5225 (in SC)
Contact: Louise Ravenel, Exec Director

The Arc of SC
PO Box 61062
Columbia, SC 29260–1062
803/894–5230
Contact: Judith E. Cooper, Exec Secretary

UAP of SC
Center for Developmental Disabilities
Benson Bldg., University of South Carolina
Columbia, SC 29208
803/777–4839
Contact: Richard Ferrante, Director

PRO Parents
2712 Middleburg Drive, Suite 102
Columbia, SC 29204
803/779–3859 (V/TDD)
800/759–4776 (in SC) (V/TDD)
Contact: Colleen Lee, Program Director

Down Syndrome Association of the Lowcountry
Box 12905
Charleston, SC 29422
803/795–9262
Contact: Dr. Elizabeth S. Pilcher

South Carolina Down Syndrome Conference
Box 50466
Columbia, SC 29250
803/256–7394
Contact: Kay I. Richardson

SOUTH DAKOTA

Education Program Assistant Manager
Office of Special Education
700 Governor's Drive
Pierre, SD 57501–2293
605/773–4478
Contact: Barb Lechner

South Dakota Advocacy Services
610 Kansas City St., Suite 200A
Rapid City, SD 57701
605/342–3808
800/658–4782 (in SD)
Contact: Dianna L. Marshall, Director

The Arc of South Dakota
421 S. Pierre Street

Pierre, SD 57501–0220
605/224–8211
800/870–1272
Contact: John Stengle, Exec Director

SD University Affiliated Program
University of South Dakota
School of Medicine
Vermillion, SD 57069
605/677–5311
800/658–3080 (V/TDD)
Contact: Judy Struck, Acting Exec Director

SD Parent Connection
3701 W 49th St., Ste 200B
PO Box 84813
Sioux Falls, SD 57118
605/335–8844 (V/TDD)
800/640–4553 (in SD) (V/TDD)

Parent to Parent, Inc.
1825 S. Minnesota
Sioux Falls, SD 57105
605/334–3119
800/658–5411 (in SD)

People with Down Syndrome
1409 N. 1st Street
Aberdeen, SD 57401
605/229–4924
Contact: Robert Johnson

TENNESSEE

Special Education Programs
Department of Education
132 Cordell Hull Building
Nashville, TN 37243–0380
615/741–2851
Contact: Joseph Fisher. Asst Commissioner

TN Protection and Advocacy, Inc.
PO Box 121257
Nashville, TN 37212
615/298–1080
800/342–1660 (in TN)

The Arc of TN
1805 Hayes Street, Suite 100
Nashville, TN 37203
615/327–0294
Contact: Roger Blue, Exec Director

Boling Center for Developmental Disabilities
University of Tennessee, Memphis
711 Jefferson Avenue

Memphis, TN 38105
901/528–6511
Contact: Clyn P. McKellar, EdD.

Support and Training for Exceptional Parents (STEP)
1805 Hayes Street, Suite 100
Nashville, TN 37203
615/639–0125
800/280–7837 (in TN)
Contact: Nancy Diehl, Program Director

Parents Encouraging Parents (PEP) Program
525 Cordell Hull Building
Nashville, TN 37247
615/741–7353

Down Syndrome Support Group of South Central Tennessee
1117 Whitney Drive
Columbia, TN 38401
615/381–6360
Contact: Michaelle Rhodes

Down But Not Out
200 Royal Oak Drive
Blountville, TN 37617
615/323–0944
Contact: Kim Wise

Down Syndrome Association of Memphis, Inc.
4701 Knight Arnold
Memphis, TN 38118
901/763–4007
Contact: Janie Morgret

Down Parent's Association, Inc.
Box 120832
Nashville, TN 37212
615/373–2106
Contact: JoAnne Drumwright

Down Syndrome Awareness Group of East Tennessee
111 Chestnut Hill Road
Oak Ridge, TN 37830
615/483–3890
Contact: Judith C. Larson

TEXAS

Special Education Programs
Education Agency
1701 North Congress Avenue, Room 5–120
Austin, TX 78701

512/463–9414
Contact: Al Stewart, Coordinator

Early Childhood Intervention Program
1100 West 49th Street
Austin, TX 78756
512/502–4900
Contact: Mary Elder, Exec Director

Advocacy, Inc.
7800 Shoal Creek Blvd., Suite 171–E
Austin. TX 78757
512/454–4816
800/252–9108 (in TX)
Contact: James Comstock-Galagan, Exec
Director

The Arc of TX
1600 W 38th St., #200
Austin, TX 78731
512/454–6694
800/252–9729
Contact: Libby Doggett, Exec Director

Partnerships for Assisting Texans with
Handicaps (PATH)
1090 Longfellow Drive, Suite B
Beaumont, TX 77706–4889
409/898–4684
800/866–4726 (in TX)
Contact: Janice Meyer, Director

Pilot Parents
2818 San Gabriel
Austin, TX 78705
512/476–7044
Contact: Elaine St. Marie

Down Syndrome Support Group of Central Texas
106 Champion Drive
Austin, TX 78734
512/261–4259
Contact: Cecilia Pazderny

Down's Circle
517 Coral Place
Corpus Christi, TX 78411
512/851–1216
Contact: Bess Althaus Graham

Down Syndrome Guild
Box 821174
Dallas, TX 75382–1174
214/239–8771
Contact: Minnie Blackwell

Down Syndrome Partnership of Tarrant
County
259 Bailey Street
Ft. Worth, TX 76107
817/877–1474
Contact: Kim Marshall

Down Syndrome Association of Houston
PO Box 303
Houston, TX 77001-0303
713/682-7237

BUDS
5302 Lawndale
San Angelo, TX 76903–1110
915/655–9037
Contact: Pam & Stephen Rabb

UTAH

At Risk and Special Education Services
State Office of Education
250 East 500 South
Salt Lake City, UT 84111–3204
801/538–7706
Contact: Steven J. Kukic, Director

Special Education Services Unit
State Office of Education
250 East Fifth South
Salt Lake City, UT 84111
801/538–7708
Contact: John Killoran, 619 Coordinator

Legal Center for People with Disabilities
455 East 400 South, Suite 201
Salt Lake City, UT 84111
801/363–1347
800/662–9080 (in UT) (V/TDD)
Contact: Phyllis Geldzahler, Exec Director

The Arc of Utah
455 East 400 South, Suite 300
Salt Lake City, UT 84111
801/364–5060
800/371–5060 (in UT)
Contact: Ray Behle, Exec Director

Developmental Center for Handicapped
Persons
Utah State University, UMC 6800
Logan, UT 84322–6800
801/750–1981
Contact: Marvin Fifield, Director

Utah Parent Center
2290 East, 4500 South, Suite 110
Salt Lake City, UT 84117
801/272-1051
800/468-1160
Contact: Helen Post, Director

Utah Down Syndrome Foundation
PO Box 69 WSU
Ogden, UT 84408-0069
801/392-9553
Contact: Patty Hatch

Up with Downs
4037 Foothill Drive
Provo, UT 84604
801/225-1929
Contact: Brenda Winegar

VERMONT

Special Education Unit, Dept of Education
120 State Street
Montpelier, VT 05620-2703
802/828-3141
Contact: Kathleen Andrews, Preschool Coordinator

Division of Children with Special Needs
Department of Health
PO Box 70
Burlington, VT 05402
802/863-7338
Contact: Beverly MacCarty, Part H Coordi-
nator

Vermont DD Law Project
12 North Street, PO Box 1367
Burlington, VT 05402
802/863-2881
Contact: Judy Dickson, Director

Citizen Advocacy, Inc.
Champlain Mill, Box 37
Winooski, VT 05404
802/655-0329
Contact: Katherine Lenk, Director

Vermont ARC
Champlain Mill #37
Wirooski, VT 05404
802/655-4014
Contact: Joan Sylvester

Center for Developmental Disabilities
The University Affiliated Program of
Vermont

499C Waterman Building
University of Vermont
Burlington, VT 05405-0160
802/656-4031
Contact: Wayne L. Fox, Director

VT Parent Information Center
Chace Mill
1 Mill Street
Burlington, VT 05401
802/658-5315 (V/TT)
800/639-7170 (in VT)
Contact: Connie Curtin, Director

Parent to Parent Program
69 Champlain Mill
1 Main Street
Winooski, VT 05404
802/655-5290
Contact: Nancy DiVenere

VIRGINIA

Office of Special Education Services
Department of Education
PO Box 2120
Richmond, VA 23216-2120
804/225-2933

Infant and Toddler Program
Department of Mental Health, Mental Re-
tardation & Substance Abuse Services
PO Box 1797
Richmond, VA 23214
804/786-3710
Contact: Anne Lucas, Part H Coordinator

Department for Rights of Virginians with
Disabilities
James Monroe Building
101 North 14th Street, 17th Floor
Richmond, VA 23219
804/225-2042 (V/TDD)
800/552-3962 (in VA)
Contact: Margaret C. Hager, Director

The Arc of Virginia
6 North 6th Street
Richmond, VA 23219
804/649-8481
Contact: Steve K. Waldron, Exec Director

Virginia Institute for Developmental Disabilities
Virginia Commonwealth University
301 West Franklin Street, Box 3020
Richmond, VA 23284-3020

804/225–3876
Contact: Fred P. Orelove, Exec Director

Parent Educational Advocacy Training Center (PEATC)
Courthouse Plaza II
10340 Democracy Lane, Suite 206
Fairfax, VA 22031
703/691–7826
800/869–6782
Contact: Cherie Takemoto, Director

Parent to Parent of Virginia
Family and Children's Service
1518 Willow Lawn Drive
Richmond, VA 23230
804/282–4255
Contact: Elizabeth Fletcher, Coordinator

Parents of Down Syndrome of Shenandoah Valley
271 Branson Spring Road
Clearbrook, VA 22624
703/665–1968
Contact: Diane Brown

Down Syndrome Association of Greater Richmond
PO Box 24004
Richmond, VA 23224
804/225–3875
Contact: Pam Barton

Down Syndrome Association of Roanoke
PO Box 4683
Roanoke, VA 24015
703/774–1975
Contact: Susan J. Cloeter

Parents of Children with Down Syndrome of Northern VA
6111 Roxbury Avenue
Springfield, VA 22152
703/451–6328
Contact: Judy Farabaugh

Tidewater Down Syndrome Support Group
1828 Roves Lane
Virginia Beach, VA 23464
804/479–3713
Contact: Nancy McCullough

VIRGIN ISLANDS

State Office Early Childhood Education
Special Education/Dept of Education
44–46 Kongens Gade

St. Thomas, VI 00802
809/776–5802
Contact: Wanda Hamilton, State Coordinator

Division of Maternal and Child Health
Crippled Children's Services
Department of Health
Knud Hansen Complex
St. Thomas, VI 00802
809/776–3580
Contact: Patricia Adams, Program Director

Virgin Island Advocacy Agency
7A Whim, Suite #2
Fredericksted, St. Croix, VI 00840
809/772–1200
Contact: Camille Ayala-Walker, Exec Director

Inter-Island Parent Coalition
PO Box 4402 Christiansted
St. Croix, VI 00802
809/778–2275

WASHINGTON

Office of Superintendent of Public Instruction
Old Capitol Bldg., PO Box 7200
Olympia, WA 98504–7200
206/753–0317
Contact: Michael Conn-Powers, Coordinator

Birth to Six Planning Project
Department of Social & Health Services
PO Box 45201
Olympia, WA 98504–5201
206/586–2810
Contact: Sandy Loerch, Part H Coordinator

WA Protection & Advocacy System
1401 East Jefferson
Seattle, WA 98122
206/324–1521
Contact: Mark Stroh, Exec Director

The Arc of Washington State
1703 East State Street
Olympia, WA 98506
206/357–5596

Child Development and Mental Retardation Center
University of Washington

Seattle, WA 98195
206/543-2832
Contact: Michael Guralnick, Director

Parents are Vital in Education (PAVE)
6316 South 12th Street
Tacoma, WA 98465
206/565-2266 (V/TT)
800/572-7368 (in WA)
Contact: Lynne Leeper, Project Coordinator

Parent-to-Parent Support Programs
10550 Lake City Way, NE Suite A
Seattle, WA 98125-7752
206/948-7322
800/821-5927 (in WA)
Contact: Linda Williams, State Director

Up-Side-Downs of Grays Harbor
508 N. M Street
Aberdeen, WA 98520
206/532-6385
Contact: Anna Jean McDaniel

Children with Special Health Care Needs
3020 Rucker Avenue
Suite 200
Everett, WA 98201
206/339-5240
206/339-5216

Down Syndrome Outreach
3778 Aldergrove Road
Ferndale, WA 98248
206/366-3728
206/366-1004

Moms with Kids with Down Syndrome
6140 Capital Blvd.
Suite 632
Olympia, WA 98501
206/352-1126
Contact: Susan Atkins

Down Syndrome Community Family
Group
815 N. Third Street
Renton, WA 98055
206/255-6826
Contact: Pam Wilson

Down Syndrome Community
1720 NE 105th Street
Seattle, WA 98125
206/527-2496
Contact: Nicholas Kappes

Spokane Center of Parents with Down
Syndrome
N. 10212 Sundance Drive
Spokane, WA 99208
509/467-0192
Contact: Tami Falkner

PRIDE Program
Clark College
1800 E. McLoughlin Blvd
Vancouver, WA 98663
206/699-0394
Contact: Nancy Warren/Judy Marick

Yakima Down Syndrome Parent Support
Group
2811 Tieton Drive
Yakima, WA 98902
509/575-8160
509/575-8921
Contact: Susie Ball

DS Society of the Olympic Peninsula
10569 Sirocco Circle, NW
Silverdale, WA 98383
206/698-9483
206/698-9459
Contact: Marcia Rubenstein

Touchstones
6721 5th Ave., S
Seattle, WA 98118
206/721-0867 (V/TYY)

STOMP-Specialized Training of Military
Parents
12208 Pacific Hwy SW
Tacoma, WA 98499
800/298-3543 (Voice)
206/588-1741

WEST VIRGINIA

Preschool Disabilities
Office of Special Education Programs &
Assurances
Capitol Complex, Bldg. 6, Room 304
Charleston, WV 25305
304/558-2696
Contact: Carol Williams

Early Intervention Program
Office of Maternal and Child Health
Bureau of Public Health
1116 Quarrier Street
Charleston, WV 25301

304/558–3071
Contact: Pamela Roush, Director

Protection and Advocacy Agency
Litton Bldg., 4th Floor
1207 Quarrier Street
Charleston, WV 25301
304/346–0847 (V/TDD)
800/950–5250 (in WV)
Contact: Linda Leasure, Exec Director

Arc of WV
16 Echo Terrace
Wheeling, WV 26003
304/277–1466
Contact: Brent Bush, President

University Affiliated Center for
Developmental Disabilities (UACDD)
Airport Research & Office Park
955 Hartman Run Road
Morgantown, WV 26505
304/293–4692
Contact: Sherry Wood-Shuman, Director

WV Parent Training & Information Project
(WVPTI)
104 E. Main St.
Clarksburg, WV 26301
304/624–1436 (V/TT)
800/281–1436 (in WV)
Contact: Pat Habenbosch, Director

Project STEP
116 East King Street
Martinsburg, WV 25401
304/263–HELP
Contact: Carol Tamara, Director

Mid-Ohio Valley Down Syndrome Association
Rt. 2 Box 457
Winding Road
Parkersburg, WV 26101
304/428–2156
Contact: Sheila Pursley

WISCONSIN

Early Childhood: Exceptional Educational
Needs Program
Division for Handicapped Children &
Pupil Services
Department of Public Instruction
PO Box 7841
Madison, WI 53707

608/266–6981
Contact: Jenny Lange, Program Supervisor

Division of Community Services
Department of Health & Human Services
PO Box 7851
Madison, WI 53707
608/267–3270
Contact: Susan Robbins, Birth to 3 Coordinator

WI Coalition for Advocacy
16 North Caroll Street, Suite 400
Madison, WI 53703
608/267–0214
Contact: Lynn Breedlove, Exec Director

Waisman Center UAP
University of Wisconsin
1500 Highland Avenue
Madison, WI 53705–2280
608/263–5940
Contact: Terrence R. Dolan, Director

Parent Education Project of Wisconsin, Inc.
2192 South 60th Street
West Allis, WI 53219
414/328–5520
800/231–8382 (in WI)
Contact: Jan Serak/Charles Price, Co-Directors

Wisconsin ARC
121 S. Hancock Street
Madison, WI 53703
608/251–9272
Contact: Jon A. Nelson

Central Wisconsin Down Syndrome Parent
Support Group
1000 N. Oak, Peds 1A 329
Marshfield, WI 54449
715/387–5228
Contact: Gini Woolworth & Colleen

Down Syndrome Association of Wisconsin,
Inc.
PO Box 23384
Milwaukee, WI 53223
414–355–1404
Contact: Joan B. Balliet

SW Wisconsin Parents of DS Persons
18716 W. Mound Road
Platteville, WI 53818
608/348–8906
Contact: Connie Powers

Down Syndrome Association of Wisconsin
Dells
2755 N. 75th Street
Wauwatosa, WI 53210
414/453-7337
Contact: Nancy VanValkenburgh

WYOMING

Department of Health
Herschler Bldg. 1st Floor West
122 West 25th Street
Cheyenne, WY 82002-0050
307/777-5246
Contact: Kathy Emmons, Childrens Service Manager

Division of Developmental Disabilities
Department of Health
Herschler Building, 1st Floor West
122 West 25th St.
Cheyenne, WY 82002
307/777-6972 (V/TT)
Contact: Mitch Brauchie, Part H Coordinator

Wyoming P&A System
2424 Pioneer Avenue, #101
Cheyenne, WY 82001
307/632-3496
800/624-7648 (in WY)
Contact: Jeanne A. Thobro, Exec Director

The Arc of Wyoming
PO Box 2161
Casper, WY 82602
307/237-9110
Contact: Scott Bergey, Exec Director

Parent Information Center
5 N. Lobban
Buffalo, NY 82384
307/684-2277
800/660-9742 (in WY)
Contact: Terri Dawson, Director

Governor's Planning Council on Developmental Disabilities
122 West 25th Street
Herschler Bldg., 4th Floor/East
Cheyenne, WY 82002
307/777-7230
800/438-5791 (in WY)
Contact: Lynda Laumgardner, Family Support Consultant

Parent Resource Center
500 S. Walsh Drive
Casper, WY 82609
307/577-0321
Contact: Marilyn Skogen

ARGENTINA

Asociacion Sindrome de Down de La Republica Argentina
Victoria Bulit
Vera 863
Buenos Aires, 1414 Argentina

Fundacion Sindrome de Down Para Su Apoyo e Integracion
Nepper 80
Villa Belgrano
5147 Cordoba Argentina

AUSTRALIA

Down Syndrome Association of New South Wales, Inc.
Box 2356
North Parramatta
N.S.W. 2151
Contact: Antonia Scott

Down Syndrome Association of Queensland
Milton, Queensland 4064
Contact: Linda Orr

Down Syndrome Association of South Australia, Inc.
24 Harrow Avenue
Magil
South Australia, 5072

BRAZIL

Up, Down! Association
Rua Alexandre Herculano75
Santos, 11050
Sao Paulo
Contact: Dr. Ruy Do Amaral Pupo

Centro de Informacao & Pesquisa da Sindrome de Down
Ave Briz, Faria Lima 16984
Andar Cep. 01452
Sao Paulo

CANADA

Ups and Downs
2803 Canmore Rd., NW

Calgary, Alberta T2M 4J7
Contact: Dr. Kelly Moynihan

Squamish Community Services Society
Box 877 Squamesh
British Columbia, V0N 3G0
Contact: Liz Wood

Early Intervention Program
65 Brunswick St., #352
Fredericton
New Brunswick, E3B 1G5
Contact: Linda Beebe

Down Syndrome Association of Hamilton
Rt. 7 Brantford
Ontario N3T 5L9
Contact: Murray MacDonald

Halton Down Syndrome Association
Box 93037
Headon Postal Outlet
Burlington, Ontario L7M 4A3
Contact: John Murray

Friends
367 Wellington Street, W.
Chatham Ontario N7M 1K2
Contact: Kimberly Bossy

Quinte Down Syndrome Parent Support
Group
Box 114, 98 Fourth Street
Deseronto Ontario K0K 1X0 Canada
Contact: Mary M.J. Tinney

Nipissing Down Syndrome Society
Box 316
North Bay Ontario P1B 9N4
Contact: Rheal Thorn

Parents of Down Syndrome
428 Sundial Drive
Orillia Ontario L3V 4A6
Contact: Brenda Morris

Down Syndrome Association of York Region
1111 Davis Dr, Ste 30–345
Newmarket Ontario, L4C 5Y8
Contact: S. Smith

Down Syndrome Association of Ontario
19 Royal Birkdale Lane
Thornhill Ontario, L3T 1V1
Contact: Lynda Langdon

Up About Down
2091 W. Grand Court
Windsor Ontario, N9E 1G7
Contact: Nancy Buress

Quebec Down Syndrome Association
Montreal Children's Hospital
2300 Tupper Avenue
Montreal Quebec, H3H 1P3
Contact: J.F. Lemay, M.D.

COLUMBIA

Corporacion Sindrome de down
Calle 119A #53–48
Bogota, Colombia

COMMONWEALTH OF THE NORTHERN MARIANA ISLANDS

Special Education, Public School System
PO Box 1370 CK
Saipan, Mariana Islands 96950
011 (670) 322–9956/9590
Contact: Barbara T. Rudy, Coordinator

Early Childhood Education
Public School System
PO Box 1370
Saipan, Mariana Islands 96950
011 (670)322–9956/9590
Contact: Suzanne Lizama, Coordinator

Catholic Social Services
PO Box 745
Saipan, Mariana Islands 96950
011 (670)234–6981
Contact: Richard D. Shewman, Exec Director

ENGLAND

Down Syndrome Association
155 Mitcham Road
London, SW17 9PG
Contact: Anna Khan

HONG KONG

Hong Kong Down Syndrome Association, Ltd.
Box 4116
Hong Kong
Contact: Annie L.F. Tse

Watchdog Early Learning and Development Center
Ground Floor
12 Borrett Road

Hong Kong
Contact: Maryke DeWolf

IRELAND

Down Syndrome Association of Ireland
5 Fitzwilliam Place
Dublin 2
01–676–9255
01–676–9259
Contact: Joseph E. Greevy

INDIA

Parents of Down Syndrome
Hill Road Clinic
102 B Rizui Palace
Opp New Talkies, Bandra
Bombay 400050
Contact: Dr. Errol Rebello

ISRAEL

YATED
47 Gaza Street
Jerusalem 92383
Contact: Rachel Dotan

ITALY

Associazione Bambini Down
Viale Delle Milizie, 106
Roma 00192
Contact: Giampaolo Muti

JAPAN

Niwa Yoshiko
10–901 Senteur Nakagawa
9–2 Chome Nakagawa
Kohoku-Ku
Yokohama, 223

MALAYSIA

Kiwanis Down's Syndrome Centre
59 Jalan Gasing
Petaling Jaya
Selangor, 46000

MEXICO

Asociacion Mexicana de Sindrome de
   Down
Selva 4, Insurgentes Cuicuilco
Delegacion Coyoacan
04530 Mexico, D.F.

Down Association of Monterrey
20 De Noviembre Sur 846
Monterrey, N.L.

Fundacion Down de la Laguna
Avenida Morelos No. 43 Ote
Torreon, Coah 27000

NETHERLANDS

Stichting Down's Syndrome
Bovenboersewegf 41
Wanneperveen, NL-7946AL

NIGERIA

The Down's Syndrome Society of Nigeria
FE-50 Zoo Road, Box 10290
Kano, Nigeria
Contact: Abba Ibrahaim Bello

SOUTH AFRICA

Down Syndrome Association Natal
Box 70048 Overport
Durban 4067
Contact: Mrs. Barbara Higgins

SCOTLAND, U.K.

Scottish Down's Syndrome Association
158/160 Balgreen Road
EH11 3AU
Edinburgh
Contact: Alison McGiluray

SPAIN

Fundacio Catalana Sindrome de Down
Valencia 231
Barcelona 08007
Contact: Mrs. Montserrat Trueta

Fundacion Sindrome de Down de Cant-
   abria
Avda. de General Davila
24–A, 1.O.C.
39005 Santander

Asoc. Sindrome de Down de Baleares
Carretera Palma-Alcudia
Km. 7,5
07141 Marratxi
Baleares

SAUDI ARABIA

Help Center
PO Box 1049
Jeddah 21431

Index